Acknowledgements

The American Red Cross First Aid—Responding to Emergencies course, textbook, and instructor's manual were developed and produced through a joint effort of the American Red Cross and the Mosby-Year Book Publishing Company.

Members of the Development Team at American Red Cross national headquarters responsible for developing this instructor's manual included: M. Elizabeth Buoy-Morrissey, M.P.H., Development Team Leader and Writer; Lawrence D. Newell, Ed.D., NREMT-P, and S. Elizabeth White, M.A.Ed., ATC, Writers and Instructional Designers; Martha F. Beshers and Joan H. Timberlake, Editors; and Jane Moore, Desktop Publisher.

The following American Red Cross national headquarters Health and Safety paid and volunteer staff provided guidance and review: John M. Malatak, Ph.D., Assistant Director; Frank Carroll, Manager, Development; Jean M. Wagaman, Associate, Operations; Israel Zuniga, Associate, Development; Marian F. H. Kirk and O. Paul Stearns, III, Analysts, Development; and Stephen Silverman, Ed.D., National Volunteer Consultant, Development.

The Mosby-Year Book Production team included: David T. Culverwell, Publisher; Richard A. Weimer, Executive Editor; Claire Merrick, Senior Editor; Patricia Gayle May, Project Manager; Mary Cusick Drone, Production Editor.

Special thanks go to Becky Kennedy Koch, M.Ed., ATC, The Ohio State University, Columbus, Ohio, for assistance in writing; to Janet Head, RN, M.S., and Michael French, B.S., Kirksville College of Osteopathic Medicine, Kirksville, Missouri, for writing the test bank questions; and to Tom Lochhaas, Developmental Editor.

Guidance and review was also provided by members of the American Red Cross First Aid Advisory Committee:

Sergeant Ray Cranston, Chairperson, Farmington Hills Police Department, Farmington Hills, Michigan

Kathleen C. Oberlin, Subcommittee Chairperson, Specialist, Health and Safety ,Western Operations Headquarters, American Red Cross, Burlingame, California

Ann E. Graziadei, Ed.S., A.T., C., Department of Physical Education and Recreation, Gallaudet University, Washington, D.C.

Candace Key Gregg, M.S., E.M.T., Director of Health and Safety, American Red Cross Tuscaloosa County Chapter, Tuscaloosa, Alabama

Stanley Henderson, M.S.Ed., Assistant Professor, Department of Health and Safety, Indiana State University, Terre Haute, Indiana

Sam A. Lybarger, Ed.S., Safety Professional III, Reynolds Electrical and Engineering, Las Vegas, Nevada

Mary M. Newman, Emergency Medical Services Consultant, Carmel, Indiana

Donna Palmieri, Manager, Safety Services, American Red Cross Southeastern, Pennsylvania Chapter, Philadelphia, Pennsylvania

David C. Wiley, Ph.D., Assistant Professor, Department of Health, Physical Education and Recreation, Southwest Texas State University, San Marcos, Texas

Peter C. Wolk, Ed.M., J.D., Volunteer Instructor, National Capital Chapter, and Attorney, Dow, Lohnes and Albertson, Washington, D.C.

Contents

Contents

Contents

Part A: Administration

1 INTRODUCTION

This manual is intended to serve as a resource for instructors of the American Red Cross First Aid—Responding to Emergencies course. Information and teaching suggestions are provided to help you teach the course effectively, maintaining Red Cross standards. You should be familiar with the material in the *American Red Cross First Aid—Responding to Emergencies* textbook (Stock No. 650005) and in this instructor's manual before you teach the course.

Purpose of the Course

The purpose of the American Red Cross First Aid—Responding to Emergencies course is to provide the citizen responder with the knowledge and skills necessary in an emergency to help sustain life, reduce pain, and minimize the consequences of injury or sudden illness until professional medical help arrives.

The course content and activities will prepare participants to recognize emergencies and make appropriate decisions for first aid care. The course teaches the first aid skills the citizen responder will need in order to act as the first link in the emergency medical services (EMS) system.

This course includes an emphasis on prevention of injuries and illness, with a focus on personal safety. Using a healthy lifestyles awareness inventory, participants will assess their environment and personal habits to reduce their own risk of injury and illness.

Course Objectives

At the conclusion of this course, participants should be able to—

- Explain how the EMS system works and the citizen responder's role in the EMS system.
- Explain what happens in the body if one or more body systems fail to function properly.
- Identify and care for choking and other breathing emergencies.
- Identify the major risk factors for cardiovascular disease, and injury, and describe how to control them.

- Recognize the signals of a possible heart attack, and describe how to care for someone who is experiencing persistent chest pain.
- Identify the signals of cardiac arrest, and demonstrate how to provide cardiopulmonary resuscitation (CPR) until advanced emergency medical care arrives.
- Identify life-threatening bleeding, and demonstrate how to control it.
- Identify the signals of shock, and describe how to minimize the effects of shock.
- Identify the signals of various soft tissue and musculoskeletal injuries, and demonstrate how to care for them.
- Identify the signals of medical emergencies, including poisoning and heat and cold emergencies, and describe both general and specific care for medical emergencies.
- Describe when and how to move a victim in an emergency situation.

Authorized American Red Cross instructors may award course completion certificates to participants who meet the course completion requirements.

Purpose and Format of the Instructor's Manual

This instructor's manual contains all information necessary for conducting the American Red Cross First Aid—Responding to Emergencies course, as suggested in the lesson plans.

"Part A: Administration" contains information needed to conduct the course. It provides a course overview, describes course organization, tells how to set up and teach the course, explains how to run practice sessions, gives requirements for successful course completion, and describes what to do after the course is completed.

"Part B: Teaching Tools" includes the course outline, and the lesson plans. The course outline provides a summary of suggested activities for each lesson plan and totals the running time for the various parts of the course. The lesson plans are designed to be used as a guide for course delivery.

The Appendixes include teaching aids, final examinations, a test bank, and evaluation forms.

Instructor's Responsibilities

Your responsibilities as an authorized Red Cross First Aid—Responding to Emergencies instructor are to—

- Be familiar with the course materials and know how to use them effectively.
- Plan, coordinate, and manage the course in conjunction with the local Red Cross unit.
- Inform participants of evaluation procedures and course completion requirements.
- Create a nonthreatening environment that is conducive to the achievement of course objectives.
- Adapt your teaching approaches to the experience and ability of participants, while still enabling them to meet the course objectives.
- Be prepared to answer participants' questions, or know where to find the answers.
- Provide for the health and safety of participants by ensuring that—
  a. Manikins have been properly cleaned according to the recommendations in Appendix A.
  b. Participants are aware of health precautions and guidelines concerning the transmission of infectious diseases and their physical ability to perform the first aid skills.
  c. Participants know they should consult you if they have concerns about their physical ability to perform the first aid skills.
  d. The classroom and practice areas are free of hazards.
- Be able to demonstrate all the skills taught in this course.
- Supervise participants while they are practicing the skills.
- Provide participants with constructive feedback as they learn the skills and go through the decision-making process required by the scenarios.
- Evaluate participants' performance of skills.
- Identify participants who are having difficulty mastering the course materials, and develop effective strategies for remediation.
- Administer and score the final written examination.
- Ensure that course completion requirements are met.
- Issue course completion certificates.
- Submit completed course records and reports to Red Cross representatives within the time required by the local Red Cross unit.
- Use the information on risk factors included in this course as a way to introduce other Red Cross courses. Information on other Red Cross courses is printed on the inside back cover of the textbook.
- Be familiar with the Red Cross publications, brochures, decals, and emblems available from your local Red Cross unit.

- Not smoke or show other unhealthy habits when working with participants.
- Identify potential instructor candidates and refer them to the appropriate Red Cross representative.
- Abide by the obligations in the Instructor Agreement and, if applicable, the Authorized Provider Agreement.

Appendix O—Administrative Terms and Procedures, defines many of the terms and procedures you need to know as a Red Cross instructor.

2 COURSE DESIGN

Course Content

In order to achieve the purpose of this course, the content provides consistent guidelines that will enable a citizen to provide appropriate care, regardless of the type of emergency. The course stresses the basic steps to follow in an emergency, beginning with the most important—**the decision to act**—and helps participants confront their fears of stepping forward to give assistance.

Course content clarifies **when** and **how** to call the Emergency Medical Services system, eliminating confusion that often causes delays in obtaining more highly trained medical care. It also emphasizes the need for rapid medical assistance in life-threatening emergencies.

Course activities build sequentially on material covered. Focusing on prevention, as well as first aid, course activities motivate participants to evaluate their lifestyles and set personal goals for improved health.

The course is designed to allow for flexibility in delivery. You should not modify course content, but you have flexibility to select teaching methods to meet the needs and interests of participants as long as they can meet the course objectives. You may wish to emphasize certain aspects of the content. For example, if you teach the course in a high school, you might emphasize prevention of injuries that are most common in that age group. If time allows, you may also wish to teach additional Red Cross courses in conjunction with this First Aid—Responding to Emergencies course. American Red Cross courses such as CPR: Infant and Child, CPR: Basic Life Support for the Professional Rescuer, or Basic Water Safety are excellent adjuncts.

Course Components

The course components include a participant textbook, a video, transparencies, two written examinations, and a computerized test bank. A description of each component follows.

Textbook

The participant's textbook serves as a learning tool to use before, during, and after the course. It contributes to elimination of lengthy lectures and explanations, and should make class discussions more meaningful. Most lessons include out-of-class reading assignments from the textbook to prepare participants for the class activities.

The textbook has been designed to facilitate learning and understanding of the material. It includes the following features:

- **Learning Objectives**
  At the beginning of each chapter is a list of objectives that describe what participants should be able to do after reading the chapter and participating in class activities.
- **Key Terms**
  Following the objectives is a list of defined key terms that the participant needs to know in order to understand chapter content. A few key terms are listed in more than one chapter because they are essential to understanding the material presented in each. The pronunciation of certain medical and anatomical terms is provided, and a pronunciation guide is included in the glossary. In the chapter, key terms are printed in boldface the first time they appear.
- **"For Review"**
  This section indicates information the participant should already be familiar with in order to more easily understand the chapter.
- **Sidebars**
  Articles called sidebars enhance the information in the main body of the text. They appear in all chapters on a lavender background. They present a variety of material ranging from historical information and accounts of actual events to everyday application of the chapter's information. This design feature helps make text material more interesting. American Red Cross course completion requirements do not require participants to know any information presented in the sidebars.
- **Figures**
  Photographs and illustrations reinforce concepts and information in the chapter.
- **Tables**
  Tables, on a blue background, are included in many chapters. They concisely summarize important concepts and aid studying.
- **Application Questions**
  Application questions, designated with a "Q" inside a yellow bar, challenge participants to apply the information they have learned and build a solution. Participants should answer the application questions as they read the chapter. The answers to these questions are in each chapter, after the summary.
- **Study Questions**
  Also at the end of each chapter, on a rose-colored background, is a series of questions designed to aid retention and understanding of the content. Space is left after the questions to allow participants to write most answers directly in the textbook.

Completing these questions will help participants evaluate how well they understand the material and help prepare them for the final written exam. The answers are in Appendix A of the textbook.

Direct participants how to use the study questions. Tell them to answer as many questions as they can without referring back to the chapter, then review the information covering any questions they were unable to answer and try them again. They should check their responses with the answers in Appendix A. If an answer is incorrect, they should reread that part of the chapter. If, after rereading the information, they still do not understand, they should ask you to help.

- **Skill Sheets**
  Illustrated skill sheets at the end of certain chapters give step-by-step directions for performing specific skills. The skill sheets are designed to aid participants in their review and practice of the skills taught in this course. There is a band of blue on the outside edge of each skill sheet page to help locate them quickly.
- **Appendixes**
  Appendixes at the end of the textbook provide the answers to the study questions and additional information on certain topics. For example, Appendix B gives detailed information on first aid and disease transmission; Appendix C discusses the protection offered citizen responders by Good Samaritan laws; and Appendix D contains the Healthy Lifestyles Awareness Inventory.
- **Glossary**
  The glossary defines all the key terms and other words in the text that may be unfamiliar. A guide to pronunciation is included at the front of the glossary.
- **Sources**
  The sources section includes a list of books and articles that were used as resources in writing the textbook.

Video

One video, approximately two hours long, is available for this course. The video is designed to supplement the learning experiences by providing vital information about emergency response and to set up class discussions. It includes emergency situations in real-life settings, and studio demonstrations of skills participants will learn.

Although other videos or films may be added to enhance learning, this video was specifically designed to be used with this course. Since many of the skills and practice sessions build upon each other, it is strongly recommended that you not change the order in which the video segments are shown and the skills practiced.
The order of the video segments and chapters in the textbook to which they correspond are as follows:

Course Design

Text		Video
Part One:	**Introduction**	
Chapter 1	The Citizen Responder	*Barriers to Action*
Chapter 2	Body Systems	*Understanding the Human Body* (shown as the third video)
Part Two:	**Assessment**	*Emergency Action Principles* (shown as the second video)
Chapter 3	Responding to Emergencies	*The Primary Survey* *The Secondary Survey*
Part Three:	**Life-Threatening Emergencies**	
Chapter 4	Breathing Emergencies	*The Primary Survey: Rescue Breathing* *The Primary Survey: Putting It All Together* *The Primary Survey: Obstructed Airway (Unconscious Adult)* *Obstructed Airway (Conscious Adult)*
Chapter 5	Cardiac Emergencies	*Recognizing a Heart Attack* *The Primary Survey: CPR*
Chapter 6	Bleeding	*The Primary Survey: Severe Bleeding*
Chapter 7	Shock	
Part Four:	**Injuries**	
Chapter 8	Soft Tissue Injuries	*Injuries* *Controlling Bleeding*
Chapter 9	Musculoskeletal Injuries	*Splinting*
Chapter 10	Injuries to the Head and Spine	
Chapter 11	Injuries to the Chest, Abdomen, and Pelvis	
Chapter 12	Injuries to the Extremities	

(continued on page 11)

Text		Video
Part Five:	**Medical Emergencies**	
Chapter 13	Sudden Illnesses	*Medical Emergencies*
Chapter 14	Poisoning, Bites, and Stings	
Chapter 15	Substance Misuse and Abuse	
Chapter 16	Heat and Cold Exposure	
Part Six:	**Rescues**	
Chapter 17	Reaching and Moving Victims	*Rescue Moves*
Part Seven:	**Healthy Lifestyles**	
Chapter 18	Your Guide to a Healthier Life	

Transparencies

Forty-eight full-color transparencies featuring anatomical and other key illustrations are available as a separate item. Appendix P contains a list of these transparencies.

Transparency masters are included in Appendix Q. They are designed to support the classroom instruction at your discretion. You may choose to use some of them as handouts.

Written Examinations

Two 70-question examination forms, A and B, are included in Appendix B of this manual. Give either examination A or examination B as part of the requirements for receiving an American Red Cross course completion certificate. The questions have been carefully selected from the test bank to test the participants' ability to meet the course objectives. Other questions should not be substituted.

Appendix C includes the questions contained in the computerized test bank. The questions are divided by chapter, and each question notes the chapter objective it tests. The test bank questions may be used to prepare the self-assessment quizzes as well as to prepare formal examinations for academic requirements other than those of the American Red Cross.

Computerized Test Bank

The computerized test bank package contains approximately 500 test questions. Formatted for flexibility, the test bank includes multiple-choice, true/false, matching and short answer questions. You can add, edit, or delete test items as you prepare formal examinations. Computer programs are compatible with the IBM PC, Apple IIc, and Apple IIe computers. The test bank includes aids for—

Testing

The test generator allows you to select items from the test bank manually or randomly and to add to, edit, or delete them. It is documented with a user's manual so you can create your own questions in a preset format. It includes multiple-choice, true-false, short answer, and matching options. Examinations may be saved or printed without saving. Adjustable print options allow changes to the type size and format.

Grading

The recordkeeper saves up to 250 student names and 50 tests or assignments in a format similar to that of manual gradebooks. It features automated grade-curving, weighting, and statistics on individual and class performance.

Proctor

This tutorial segment allows you to prepare examinations participants can take at their own pace, using interactive computer terminals. Proctor also grades the tests and records scores. Participants can get results immediately and have the opportunity to review any questions that were missed.

Using the Lesson Plans

Several items in the lesson plans may help you conduct the course. These include—

- Primary points.
- Activities.
- Instructor notes.
- Audiovisual aids (video, color transparencies, and transparency masters).

Primary Points

The primary points represent the information from the lesson most important for the participants to understand. They summarize the critical material that the participants should have abstracted from reading the assigned chapter. They also represent the information needed to achieve the objectives, successfully complete the skill checks, and pass the final written examination.

You may cover these points using a variety of teaching methods. They are not meant to be points that you merely lecture about, though lecture is an acceptable teaching method. You can cover many of them during the class activities. Refer to the *American Red Cross Instructor Candidate Training Participant's Manual* (Stock No. 329741) to review various teaching strategies and for information on using audiovisual materials.

Activities

The activities that accompany the lessons are designed to promote active participation. Active participation better enables participants to understand the concepts because they are able to immediately apply what they have learned to a real-life situation. Each lesson has at least one activity that encourages active participation.

Some lessons have activities that involve "Putting It All Together." These activities enable the participants to apply previously learned skills and knowledge. They reinforce retention of skills and knowledge that participants can apply in future lessons and in real emergencies.

Instructor Notes

Space is provided in the right hand margin for you to write notes that apply to specific areas of the lesson. You may want to use this space to write particular questions you want to ask or answers to questions included in the lesson. You may also want to write in other activities that you can use to cover the primary points and enhance participation.

Audiovisual Aids

A video, color transparencies, and transparency masters (that can also be copied and used as handouts) are available to supplement learning. Appropriate use of these items is identified in the lessons. You are encouraged to use these aids to help enhance learning.

Assignments

Assignments for the next lesson are given at the end of each lesson. Direct participants to complete the study questions as they read each chapter.

Self-Assessment Exercises

Three self-assessment exercises are built into the course. It is suggested that you use the questions from the test bank (Appendix C) to develop these exercises. Since the questions are grouped by chapter, you can select appropriate questions that test participants' abilities to meet the objectives for each chapter.

Class Activities

Class activities are varied in order to enhance learning. Much of the class time is spent in sessions involving skill practice, problem-solving, and decision-making. Class discussions and videos are designed to provide key information and to alleviate the need for lengthy lectures and demonstrations.

Skill Practice

In some of the skill practice sessions, participants will practice on one another, as well as on manikins. Practice on a "real-life" victim is important in order to give participants experience in handling a real person. However, skills that require mouth-to-mouth contact, such as rescue breathing and CPR, are practiced only on manikins.

Scenarios

As stated in Chapter 1 of this manual, appropriate response in any emergency requires someone to make decisions. Scenarios are included as part of the class activities in order to help develop participants' problem-solving and decision-making skills and to help participants practice applying the skills they have learned in simulated emergencies.

The scenarios depict a variety of emergency situations. Your role is to provide the participants with information and guide them through the decision-making process, using key questions and providing feedback.

More detailed information on the scenarios is included in the individual lesson plans in Part B of this manual.

Discussion

Guided discussion is used to reinforce the information provided by the textbook and video, and to encourage participants to apply the information in different contexts.

Course Evaluation

Appendix D contains an example of a Course Evaluation Form to be completed by participants. This evaluation, or a similar one used by your local Red Cross unit, should be given to participants when the course is completed to find out how they felt about the course. Their evaluations should be returned to your local Red Cross unit, not to Red Cross national headquarters.

Instructor Evaluation

Appendix E contains an Instructor Evaluation Form. This evaluation asks your opinion about the course materials. You are asked to complete this form the first time that you teach the course. The information will help evaluate how well the course materials work for both new and experienced instructors.

The form should be returned directly to:

American Red Cross National Headquarters
Health and Safety Course Evaluations
17th and D Streets, N.W.
Washington, DC 20006

3 SETTING UP AND RUNNING THIS COURSE

Course Participants

The majority of participants will be taking this course in an academic environment—high school, college, or university. They may be taking the course in order to fulfill employment requirements, to complete requirements for a major area of study or certification, or for personal satisfaction.

There are **no** prerequisites such as previous training in first aid for enrollment in this course.

Health Requirements for Course Participants

The American Red Cross has a responsibility to safeguard the health and safety of participants enrolled in any course of instruction. The materials and procedures for teaching this course have been written to reflect this concern.

As an American Red Cross instructor, one of your responsibilities is to protect participants from health risks. The procedures outlined in this manual are designed to—

- Limit the risk of transmission of communicable diseases.
- Limit the risk of one participant injuring another when practicing on a partner.
- Limit the risk that the strenuous activity involved in practice could cause injury or sudden illness.

When possible, prospective participants should be provided information about health requirements and safety before enrolling in the course. At the beginning of the course, participants will be instructed to read the information on health and safety (pages xx to xxi of the textbook.)

Ask participants to talk to you before the first practice session, and any subsequent practice session, if they are in doubt about whether or not they can participate in any class activity involving practice.

Persons with health conditions, such as a history of a heart attack or other heart conditions, respiratory problems, or other physical limitations, may question whether or not they should take part in the practice sessions. Suggest that these participants check with their personal physician before participating in practice sessions involving physical activity. The American Red Cross advocates that, whenever possible, participants' activity levels should be adjusted to facilitate learning and help participants meet course objectives.

Tell individuals who take the course but who cannot demonstrate the skills taught in the practice sessions that they cannot be given an American Red Cross course completion certificate. However, encourage them to participate as fully as possible. They can read the textbook, participate in decision-making scenarios, watch skill practice, and otherwise participate in class activities.

Recommended Class Size

The course outline and lesson plans have been developed for a class of approximately 20 to 25 people. If your class is larger than this, you should allow more time, or have co-instructors or instructor aides to help you (see Appendix F, Use of Instructor Aides). The number of manikins available may limit class size. Personal supervision is necessary to ensure effective practice and the safety of participants. It is important that you check to see that participants follow directions. During practice sessions, you should check that participants clean the manikins properly. If the class is too large, you may not be able to provide proper supervision or to complete class activities in the time allotted.

Classroom Environment

The classroom setting should provide a safe, comfortable, and appropriate learning environment. The room should be well-lighted and ventilated, and comfortable in temperature. The classroom should provide enough space for adequate skill practice. There should be a separate area for lectures, discussion, and examinations. If the practice area is not carpeted, provide some knee protection (folded blankets or mats) for participants or allow them to bring their own padding materials. The room should be convenient to restrooms and exits.

Participants' chairs can be arranged in rows facing the front of the classroom, but you should also consider the advantages of different seating arrangements, or of rearranging seating during the class. Semicircular or circular arrangements may make participants feel more at ease at particular times. For example, when introducing the course, it may make it easier for participants to see each other clearly while introducing themselves. When participants are taking the final written examination, it may be better to have the chairs arranged to allow everyone as much space as possible to reduce distractions. When participants are practicing, they may need to push their desks against the wall to gain more floor space.

Whatever seating arrangement you select, make sure that all participants are seated so that they can adequately see the monitor or screen when you use audiovisual materials or present skill demonstrations.

To prevent injury, participants should not be asked to move heavy equipment and furniture. If their help is required, be sure that two or more participants move heavy items and that they use proper lifting techniques.

Course Materials and Equipment

Books and Other Course Components

The following items can be ordered from your local Red Cross unit or from Mosby-Year Book:

- *American Red Cross First Aid—Responding to Emergencies* textbook (Stock No. 650005)
- *American Red Cross First Aid—Responding to Emergencies Instructor's Manual* (Stock No. 650010)
- *American Red Cross First Aid—Responding to Emergencies* video (Stock No. 650018)
- *American Red Cross First Aid—Responding to Emergencies Computerized Test Bank,* IBM version (Stock No. 650022)
- *American Red Cross First Aid—Responding to Emergencies Computerized Test Bank,* Apple version (Stock No. 650023)
- *American Red Cross First Aid—Responding to Emergencies Color Transparencies* (Stock No. 650012)

Course completion certificates are available only through your local Red Cross unit. They can only be awarded by authorized American Red Cross instructors. Two certificates are awarded to participants who successfully complete the course:

- *American Red Cross First Aid—Responding to Emergencies* certificate (Stock No. 653215)
- *American Red Cross Adult CPR* certificate (C-3212)

Participant's Materials

Each participant will need a textbook. For self-assessments and the written examination, each participant will need a copy of the exercise or examination and a blank answer sheet.

Instructor's Materials and Equipment

You will need a textbook, as well as this instructor's manual. If you are going to use the video, you will need a 1/2-inch videocassette player and monitor. If you are going to use overhead transparencies, you will also need an overhead projector. If you are not familiar with the equipment, make arrangements for proper instruction, and practice prior to class. All equipment should be checked to ensure that it is working properly and that you have any additional supplies, such as an extension cord and extra bulbs for the overhead projector. You may find it helpful to complete the Video Calibration Chart in Appendix H to help you locate specific video segments.

Equipment and supplies needed to teach this course are available through your local Red Cross unit. Some units may have a limited supply; therefore, it is important to be aware of your unit's reservation policies. Early planning is necessary to determine the dates and times when certain equipment and supplies will be needed. If you are dependent on your local unit for equipment and supplies, you should make contact at least several weeks in advance to ensure that you can obtain the proper equipment and supplies for each class session. A complete list of equipment and supplies needed to teach this course, including first aid supplies such as bandages and splinting devices, is in Appendix G.

Manikins

Manikins are required equipment for this course. A participant-to-manikin ratio of 2-to-1 or 3-to-1 is recommended. Use adult manikins, either full-body or torso models. All manikins should be well-maintained and working properly.

Some manikins need to be decontaminated during use. (See page 21 and Appendix A.) Some of the newer manikins have disposable plastic bags that protrude from the mouth and cover the manikin's face. Others have individual manikin faces that are applied at the time of practice and removed after an individual has practiced a skill. All manikins should be models that can be decontaminated after class according to the recommendations contained in Appendix A.

Manikin Decontamination Supplies

To decontaminate manikins during use, you will need a decontaminating solution and a large number of gauze pads. The recommended solution is 1/4 cup of liquid chlorine bleach per gallon of tap water. This solution should be made prior to each class and discarded after use. Do not use scented bleach. The perfume in these bleaches may impart a taste to the plastics.

Since some people find bleach objectionable, 70 percent alcohol (isopropanol or ethanol) is suggested as an alternative. Although alcohol can kill many bacteria and viruses, there are some that it will not kill. However, if the manikin's face is scrubbed vigorously with 70 percent alcohol and a clean gauze pad, it is highly unlikely that any infectious disease will be transmitted. For more information on selecting one of these decontaminating solutions, review the recommendations on manikin decontamination in Appendix A.

Manikin Decontamination Procedure

During practice sessions, the manikin's entire face and the inside of its mouth must be cleaned after use by each participant. Demonstrate the following procedure, telling participants that they should use this procedure to clean the manikin's face after they use the manikin.

1. Dry the manikin's face with a clean 4" x 4" gauze pad.
2. Wet a second clean gauze pad with decontaminating solution.
3. Squeeze excess solution from the pad.
4. Scrub the manikin's entire face and the inside of its mouth vigorously with the soaked pad (being careful not to tear the mouth).
5. Place the wet pad over the manikin's mouth and nose and wait 30 seconds.
6. Discard the pad and dry the manikin's face with a third clean gauze pad.

Tell participants that, in order to keep manikins' faces clean and free from dirt, they should not place manikins facedown.

Manikin Decontamination After Class

As soon as possible after the end of each class session, all manikins should be properly cleaned. Manufacturer's recommendations should be followed regarding disassembly. The parts should be scrubbed with warm soapy water, rinsed, and decontaminated with a solution of liquid household chlorine bleach and water (1/4 cup of bleach to one gallon of water). Vigorous scrubbing with soap and water is as important as scrubbing with bleach. Disposable gloves should be worn while decontaminating manikins. Detailed information on manikin decontamination is in Appendix A.

To decontaminate the manikins after class, you will need, in addition to the decontamination solution and gauze pads, a baby bottle brush, soap and water, basins or buckets, nonsterile disposable gloves, and any further supplies that may be recommended by the manikin manufacturer. The manikin's body, hair, and clothes should be washed periodically to ensure that the manikins are clean and attractive.

4 HOW TO RUN PRACTICE SESSIONS

During the practice sessions, participants are learning and perfecting skills through practice. The participants also use these skills in activities involving simulated emergency situations, or scenarios. These activities are part of the sessions entitled, "Putting It All Together."

You must decide how best to design the practice sessions to ensure success. The practice sessions should include direction and instruction, ample practice time, instructor reinforcement and corrective feedback, and encouragement.

Plan the practice sessions to reinforce the following learning objectives. Participants should be able to—

- Describe when to call EMS personnel and demonstrate how to provide all necessary information about the emergency.
- Demonstrate how to apply the emergency action principles to a specific emergency to determine the priority of care for a victim.
- Describe the priority of care for any emergency (airway, breathing, and circulation) following the survey of the scene.
- Demonstrate how to care for victims of specific emergencies.

Before each class meets, you should set up an area in the classroom where students can practice.

In general, practice sessions will include instructor-led practice and reciprocal (partner) practice. During the practice sessions, you are responsible for—

- Demonstrating and/or guiding students through a skill.
- Keeping the practice sessions running smoothly.
- Identifying errors promptly and providing corrective feedback to assist participants to improve their skills.
- Encouraging participants to improve their skills.
- Checking each student for skill competency. (See Chapter 5 of this manual.)
- Ensuring a safe practice environment and continued safety during the practice session.

Orienting Participants to Practice Sessions

Before the first manikin practice session, you should tell participants to do the following:

- Review the information on first aid and infectious disease on pages xx and xxi of the textbook. Tell participants that if they have any of the health conditions listed, they should request a separate manikin.

- Wear a minimum of jewelry to class, remembering that jewelry should be removed, as well as lipstick, chewing gum, or tobacco. Remove pens and pencils from pockets.
- Place jewelry in a safe place, such as a purse or deep pocket.
- Have clean hands.
- Refrain from smoking, using smokeless tobacco products, eating, chewing gum, or drinking during the practice sessions.

Orienting participants to the practice sessions will help them get started more quickly and practice more efficiently. Explain that they will use the skill sheets in their textbook as a guide. They will practice in groups of two or three (according to space and supplies). Some practice sessions—primary survey, secondary survey, first aid for a conscious victim with an obstructed airway, bleeding control, and splinting—require participants to practice on another participant. Others—CPR, first aid for an unconscious victim with an obstructed airway, and rescue breathing—require practice only on a manikin.

Use of Skill Sheets

A skill sheet is included for each skill that participants will practice and be checked on. You should be able to explain how to use the skill sheets.

Each skill sheet includes illustrations that show how each skill is performed. Concise directions for performing the parts of each skill are in black type next to the illustrations.

Check boxes are provided on the skill sheet for partner or instructor check off of skills. Each box can be checked after the person practicing has demonstrated the skill and can perform it correctly without any assistance. In this way, participants can recognize any deficiencies in their skill performance.

Decision points, in blue type, describe what care should be provided when certain conditions are found. For example, during the check for consciousness in the primary survey, if the victim responds, the rescuer would begin a secondary survey. However, if the victim does not respond, the rescuer would shout for help, position the victim on the back (if necessary), and open the airway, which are the next steps on the skill sheet. By reacting to various conditions, participants are able to better understand how a skill would be used in an actual emergency situation instead of memorizing seemingly unrelated sets of skills.

Practice on Another Participant

Practice on another participant has been included in order to give participants experience handling a real person. One participant acts as the victim while another gives first aid.

Participants change roles so that each person in the group has a chance to practice the skill.

Practice on a real "victim" is important, but some precautions need to be taken so participants do not get hurt:

- Horseplay can lead to injury—do not allow horseplay during the practice sessions.
- Tell participants to observe the cautions on the skill sheets.
- **Tell participants that they should not make mouth-to-mouth contact with a partner,** should not give actual rescue breaths, and should not perform abdominal thrusts or chest compressions.

Practice on a Manikin

Participants must practice on a manikin to learn the complete procedures for rescue breathing, first aid for an unconscious victim with an obstructed airway, and CPR. Participants who do not successfully demonstrate these skills on a manikin cannot receive an American Red Cross course completion certificate.

Having the manikins out at the beginning of class can help save valuable class time. If you put the manikins out before class, you should cover the faces with a shield or piece of gauze in order to keep them clean. If you choose to keep the manikins in their cases until the beginning of the practice session, allow a few minutes to get them out at the beginning of the practice session.

Reciprocal Practice

Reciprocal (partner) practice allows participants to practice skills at their own pace. For partner practice, one person performs the steps listed on the skill sheet. The partner reads the directions to the "rescuer" and observes him or her practice the skill. The partner should point out any errors to the "rescuer" so that he or she practices the skill correctly. The partner can also mark each check box as the "rescuer" demonstrates the steps correctly.

If you choose to use reciprocal practice, you should briefly demonstrate with a participant how partners can practice together using the skill sheets.

Instructor-Led Practice

Instructor-led practice, or drill, can be used as a method of speeding up skill practice. It is particularly useful for introducing new skills that build upon previously learned skills, for example, adding chest compressions to rescue breathing to perform CPR.

When you lead the practice, position the participants so that you can see them all individually. If the participants are practicing on manikins, the manikins' heads should be pointing in the same direction and the participants should be positioned in the same orientation to the manikins. If the participants are practicing on partners, this allows you to judge skill competency as well as ensure participant safety.

Read each step on the skill sheets aloud, and have participants do each step together as a group, one step at a time. For most skills, the participants should be given adequate time to continue practicing on their own.

Helping Participants to Practice Correctly

You should watch for and correct errors participants make while practicing. Try to correct problems as soon as possible so that the skill is practiced and learned correctly. While you are working closely with one participant, check others with an occasional glance. Excuse yourself briefly to correct major problems so that participants will not continue to practice incorrectly. Encourage participants to ask questions if they are unsure how to perform any part of a skill. Stay available throughout the practice session to assist participants who require your help.

A positive learning environment is important. Participants perform best when they are kept informed of their progress. When they are practicing correctly, provide positive feedback. If they are practicing incorrectly, provide corrective feedback. Before saying what they are doing wrong, tell them what they are doing correctly. Then, tactfully help them to correct their errors.

Refer them to the textbook when appropriate. Other strategies for corrective feedback include the following:

- ◆ If the error is simple, explain directly and positively how to correct the skill. Be specific when providing feedback. For example, if the participant is having trouble opening the airway, you might say, "Your hand position is good, but you should tilt the head back farther. That will open the airway."
- ◆ You may have to show the participant what he or she should be doing. For the previous example, you might have to tilt the manikin's head yourself to show the participant how far back the manikin's head should be to open the airway.
- ◆ It may help to tell the participants why they should perform a

skill in a certain way. This may help them remember to perform the skill correctly. For example, if a participant continues to forget to call for help after checking for consciousness, you might remind the participant to call for help at this point because he or she has found out that the person is unconscious, and will need someone to call EMS personnel.

- If a participant has a continuing problem with technique, carefully observe what he or she is doing. Give exact instructions for performing the technique the correct way, and lead the participant through the instructions. For example, if a participant's hand position for chest compressions is incorrect, you might guide the participant, step by step, through the procedure for finding the correct hand position.

Throughout this process, you should continue to remind the participants of what they are doing right, as well as what they are doing wrong. Use phrases like "Your compressions are very smooth, but they should be a little deeper," or "You are doing a nice job locating the pulse, but you need to feel for a pulse for a longer time to be sure that it is present or absent." Help participants focus on the "critical" aspects for each skill, that when performed incorrectly may be life-threatening. Use Appendix I to help you identify critical errors.

Physically Challenged Participants

Information on helping participants overcome physical limitations is included in Appendix J.

5 REQUIREMENTS FOR SUCCESSFUL COURSE COMPLETION

Criteria for Course Completion and Certification

To receive the two course completion certificates for the American Red Cross First Aid—Responding to Emergencies course the participant must—

- Demonstrate competency in each skill taught in the course.
- Correctly answer at least 80 percent of the final examination questions.

Participants should be told of the requirements when they enroll for the course and during the course introduction.

Evaluating Skills

Checking skill competency is an important responsibility. Making accurate and consistent judgments on skill checks enables you to fairly evaluate each participant's skills. Checking each participant's competency at demonstrating each skill enables you to—

- Identify those participants who can correctly demonstrate the skills.
- Identify those who are having difficulty demonstrating the skills, and arrange additional time for skill practice.
- Determine each participant's ability to recognize an emergency and take appropriate action.

Your judgment on whether or not a participant can competently demonstrate a skill plays a major role in maintaining the high quality of Red Cross first aid instruction. More important, the knowledge that he or she can demonstrate a skill competently will help build the participant's confidence in his or her ability to act appropriately in a real emergency.

Checking skills should not be a fearful event for the participant. These checks are best done informally for each individual. Provide participants with continual feedback on their progress during the practice sessions and help them focus on the essential skill components.

Refer to the *American Red Cross Instructor Candidate Training Participant's Manual* (Stock No. 329741) for further assistance and guidelines for evaluating skills.

How to Check Skills

You can check skills by either checking participants individually or in small groups. Unlike other Red Cross courses, this course does not mandate reciprocal practice and skills checks with a partner, followed by another evaluation of the participant's skills by the instructor.

Because of the nature of this course and the anticipated larger class size, you will need to use time wisely when checking participants' skills. If you notice a participant performing a skill appropriately while working alone, with a partner, or as part of a larger group, you may check him or her off on that skill. A formal evaluation is not necessary. However, if you are unable to observe and check off everyone during the practice time, you need to check off the remaining participants in either a formal individual evaluation or small group skills check.

If you choose to evaluate participants formally, do the following:

- Ask the participant to demonstrate the complete skill if you did not observe him or her doing so during practice. (Sometimes participants try to talk through a skill rather than perform it.)
- As the participant demonstrates the procedure, ensure that each step on the skill sheet is performed correctly.
- Give only the information that will prompt the participant as to the appropriate action to take next.
- If the participant makes a major error, stop him or her and point out the error.
- If the participant makes a minor error, allow him or her to continue. This error may be corrected by the participant as he or she proceeds through the skills.
- If the error shows a basic misunderstanding of the procedure, give corrective feedback and give the participant more time to read the textbook and practice before checking him or her again. If the error is easily corrected, recheck the participant immediately, asking him or her to correct the deficiency.
- After the participant has successfully demonstrated the skill, indicate so by marking the successful completion of the skill on the Participant Progress Log (Appendix K of this manual).

When possible, participants should be checked off on a specific skill by the end of the lesson. Should you determine that a participant cannot perform the skill properly, advise the participant that he or she needs to practice more and that you will check off the skill later. Remember that participants will have opportunities to work on these skills at other points in the course, so you will be able to check skills at a later time.

When conducting the skills check for CPR-related skills, focus on the major issues such as whether or not the participant determines absence of breathing or pulse, or airway obstruction before providing specific care. Also, make sure that the care provided was appropriate. (For example, the participant gave chest compressions only when a pulse was absent and abdominal thrusts only when airway obstruction was present.) Do not focus on minor issues such as whether or not a participant first put his or her fingers on the Adam's apple before sliding them into the groove on the side of the neck to check for a pulse. It is more important that the participant's fingers were in the right place to feel the pulse and that the participant took the time to evaluate its presence or absence before beginning chest compressions.

As another example, when giving rescue breathing, the manikin's chest should rise and fall, and breaths should be given in a reasonable period of time, i.e., every three to six seconds. The most important thing is that the rescuer breathes enough air into the lungs to see chest movement, not split-second timing. In this way, the participant will focus on the most important aspects of a skill. For further information, refer to the American Red Cross videotape, *Managing Skill Practice and Testing* (Stock No. 329460).

Written Examination

The final written examination is given at the end of the course to participants who have passed all the skill competency checks, and who want a Red Cross course completion certificate. Two 70-question examination forms, A and B, are included in Appendix B of this manual.

Either exam A or exam B should be given as part of the requirements for receiving American Red Cross completion certificates. Other examination questions should not be substituted. Participants must get 80 percent of the answers correct (56 correct out of 70 questions). Participants must not refer to their textbook when taking the examination.

Examination Security

Exam security is your responsibility. It is not recommended that participants be allowed to see the written exam before it is distributed. You should retain both the answer sheets and the exam after the participants have completed the written exam.

Criteria for Grading Participants—For American Red Cross Course Completion Only

If the participant passes all the skill competency checks but fails the written exam, you may give the alternate version of the exam after the participant has studied for a retest, or you may give the exam orally if you think that the participant's score on the written exam was low because of poor reading skills. In this case, enter each answer on the answer sheet and score the exam as usual. If the participant scores at least 80 percent on the retest, "Pass" (P) should be entered as the final grade.

The *Course Record* (Forms 6418 and 6418A) requires that you enter a grade of pass, fail, or incomplete for each participant. The information below will help you assign the correct grade:

- **"Pass" (P)** should be entered as the final grade for a participant who has passed all the skill checks and scored at least 80 percent on the final written examination.
- **"Fail" (F)** should be entered as the final grade for a participant who has not passed **all** the required skill checks and/or the final written exam and prefers not to be reexamined, or who does not pass a retest.
- **"Incomplete" (Inc)** should be entered as the final grade if the participant is unable to complete the course due to certain circumstances, such as an illness or death in the family. An "Incomplete" is given only when arrangements to complete the training have been made.

6 COURSE CONCLUSION

Awarding Certificates

Procedures for obtaining American Red Cross course completion certificates for participants in your course should be discussed with your local Red Cross unit. Be sure to follow approved procedures. You should sign the certificates before they are given to the participants. If you will be obtaining the certificates after the course is completed, you should make arrangements for getting them to the participants.

Participants will be awarded two certificates: one for American Red Cross First Aid—Responding to Emergencies, which is valid for three years, and the second for American Red Cross: Adult CPR, which is valid for one year. The stock number for the *American Red Cross First Aid—Responding to Emergencies* certificate is 653215. The stock number for the *American Red Cross Adult CPR* certificate is C–3212.

Reporting Procedures

At the conclusion of the course, the *American Red Cross Course Record* (Forms 6418 and Form 6418A) must be completed, signed, and turned in promptly to your Red Cross unit in order to receive course completion certificates. It is important that you keep a copy for your records and make a copy for the institution or organization where the course was conducted. Your local unit may require that you complete other forms such as an equipment log sheet. Problems with equipment should be reported to your Red Cross unit if you used their equipment.

Evaluation Procedures

Evaluations are beneficial in evaluating the course structure, content, instructional aids, and instructor. Several types of evaluations are recommended to be completed at the conclusion of this course.

Course Evaluation

Gaining feedback from participants is an important step in any evaluation process. It is recommended that participants have an opportunity to tell you what they thought about the course. Have them complete evaluations each time you teach this course. This information will provide you with feedback concerning the course and its instruction, and help the Red Cross maintain the high quality of the course. Make copies of Appendix D, or use your local Red Cross unit's evaluation. At the last session, give this form to each participant to be completed before they leave. Give these course evaluations to your local Red Cross unit, if required.

Instructor Evaluation

To continue to improve this course, the American Red Cross needs your help. After you teach the course the first time, use your participants' feedback to help you complete the Instructor Course Evaluation form (Appendix E). Detach and return the completed evaluation (either as a self-fold mailer, or by placing a copy in an envelope) to—

American Red Cross National Headquarters
Health and Safety Course Evaluations
17th and D Streets, N.W.
Washington, DC 20006

Write to this address also, at any time, if you wish to share any observations or suggestions that you may have about the course.

Instructor Self-Assessment

You may find it useful to use the Instructor Self-Assessment and Development evaluation in Appendix L to rate your own instructional skills.

Review Courses

Two formats for review courses for American Red Cross First Aid—Responding to Emergencies, with eligibility criteria are in Appendix M.

Part B: Teaching Tools

Course Outline: American Red Cross First Aid—Responding to Emergencies

The course described in the following lesson plans comprises 31 lessons. Each lesson includes activities that will take an estimated 45 minutes for a class of 20 to 25 participants, resulting in a total course time of 23 hours, 15 minutes.

The course has been divided into eight parts. The first seven parts correlate with the seven parts of the textbook. The eighth part includes review and the final written examination.

A complete listing of the equipment, supplies, and audiovisual aids needed for each lesson is included in Appendix G of this manual.

Parts I–III

Lesson	Content	Activity	Prior Reading Assignment	Video
1	Introduction to Course	Discussion	Preface	
2	Healthy Lifestyles	Discussion	About this Course	
3	The Citizen Responder	Discussion		✔
4	Responding to Emergencies	Discussion	1 & 3	✔
5	Body Systems	Discussion	2	✔
6	Primary/Secondary Survey I	Skill Practice: Primary Survey		✔
7	Primary/Secondary Survey II	Skill Practice: Secondary Survey		✔
8	Respiratory Emergencies I	Discussion	4	
9	Respiratory Emergencies II	Skill Practice: Rescue Breathing		✔
10	Respiratory Emergencies III	Skill Practice: Obstructed Airway		✔
11	Cardiac Emergencies I	Discussion	5	✔
12	Cardiac Emergencies II	Skill Practice: CPR		✔
13	Cardiac Emergencies III	Skill Practice: CPR		
14	Bleeding and Shock	Discussion	6 & 7	
15	Putting it All Together: Life-Threatening Emergencies I	Discussion, Scenarios		
16	Putting it All Together II	Scenarios		
Subtotal Time Parts I—III			**10 hours, 30 minutes**	

Part IV				
Lesson	**Content**	**Activity**	**Prior Reading Assignment**	**Video**
17	Injuries	Discussion	Injury Intro.	✔
18	Soft Tissue Injuries I	Skill Practice: Controlling Bleeding	8	✔
19	Soft Tissue Injuries II/ Musculoskeletal Injuries I	Discussion,	9	✔
20	Musculoskeletal Injuries II	Skill Practice: Immobilization	10 to 12	
21	Specific Injuries	Discussion	10 to 12	
22	Putting it All Together I	Discussion, Scenarios		
23	Putting it All Together II	Discussion, Scenarios		
Subtotal Time Part IV			**5 hours, 15 minutes**	
Part V				
24	Medical Emergencies	Discussion	Intro to Medical Emergencies,13, 14	✔
25	Substance Misuse and Abuse	Discussion	15	
26	Heat and Cold Exposure	Discussion	16	
27	Putting it All Together	Discussion, Scenarios		
Subtotal Time Part V			**3 hours**	
Part VI				
28	Rescue Moves	Discussion	17	✔
Subtotal Time Part VI			**45 minutes**	
Part VII				
29	Your Guide to a Healthier Life	Discussion	18	
Subtotal Time Part VII			**45 minutes**	
Part VIII				
30	Reviewing the Course	Discussion, Scenarios		
31	Final Written Examination	Examination, Evaluation		
Subtotal Time Part VIII			**1 hour, 30 minutes**	
Total Course Time			**23 hours, 15 minutes**	

Lesson 1: INTRODUCTION

Class assignment prior to this lesson: None

Length: 45 minutes

Needed: Name tags; course roster; course outline; textbook

Goal Statement: Participants will become familiar with the criteria for successful completion of this course.

INTRODUCTION TO THE COURSE

Time: 30 minutes

Instructor Notes

Activity:

1. **Instructor and Participant Introductions**
   - Introduce yourself and welcome participants to the American Red Cross First Aid—Responding to Emergencies course.
   - Have participants introduce themselves by sharing their names and their reasons for taking this course. Name tags can be used to help remember names. Ask the participants to write their full name and address on the course roster so that you can complete the *American Red Cross Course Record* (ARC 6418 and 6418A).

     Name Tags
     Course Roster
   - Give a brief description of your background and credentials. Explain that you are an American Red Cross instructor and that this course is one of many offered by the American Red Cross.
2. **Orientation to the Location**
   - Point out the locations of fire exits, telephones, restrooms, and drinking fountains, and explain building rules, if any.

- Ask participants not to eat, drink, or smoke in class. Identify the location of these designated areas.
- Ask participants to wear comfortable clothing that will enable them to participate in activities, such as the skill practices, that are conducted on the floor.

3. **Course Schedule**
   - Distribute a course outline that includes dates and times of class meetings, lesson content, and class assignments. Written tests and skill practice sessions should be clearly identified.

Course Outline

4. **Course Description**
   - Share the following goal statement with the class:
     "The purpose of this course is to train laypersons, like you, to respond appropriately to emergency situations. The course content and activities will prepare you to better recognize emergencies, make first aid decisions, and provide care with little or no first aid supplies or equipment. This course teaches the skills you will need to manage emergency situations until emergency medical services personnel arrive."
5. **How Participants Will Learn**
   - Briefly explain how the participants will learn: lectures, discussions, group activities, and skills practice. Many lessons can be supported by video and other audiovisual material. Practice sessions will involve practice with a partner and a manikin. The textbook for this course is required reading.
6. **Textbook**
   - Identify the textbook for this course: *American Red Cross First Aid—Responding to Emergencies.* Guide the participants through the textbook. Instruct the participants how best to use the textbook to master the course

Textbook

content. Point out the following features:

- Learning Objectives
- For Review
- Key Terms
- Sidebars
- Figures and Tables
- Application Questions and Answers
- Study Questions and Answers
- Skill Sheets

7. **Course Completion**
   - Describe the American Red Cross requirements for successful course completion. To receive certificates stating that the participant has successfully completed the course of instruction, the participant must—
     - Correctly demonstrate the skills taught in the course.
     - Correctly answer at least 80 percent of the final written test questions. (Participants are required to have 56 of 70 questions correct for certification.)

   Note: If there are academic requirements beyond the minimum course completion requirements set by the American Red Cross, explain them to the participants at this time.

RESPONDING TO EMERGENCIES

Time: 15 minutes

Activity:

Initiate a discussion with participants that gives them opportunities to share experiences of emergency situations involving injuries or sudden illnesses. Begin by asking if any participants have witnessed or responded to an emergency situation.

- ◆ Expect that they may describe how they or other bystanders **reacted** to an emergency and what **care** they or others gave.

- Ask how they felt about the help they provided or saw being provided.

  Note: If the participants are slow to respond or have no experiences, you should share a brief story to initiate class discussion.

  Conclude by reminding participants that they are taking this course to learn how to act appropriately and confidently in emergency situations.

Assignment:

- Read "About This Course" (pages xvii to xix in the textbook).
- Complete the Healthy Lifestyles Awareness Inventory (Appendix D in the textbook).

Lesson 2: HEALTHY LIFESTYLES

Class assignment prior to this lesson:	Read "About This Course." Complete the Healthy Lifestyles Awareness Inventory.
Length:	45 minutes
Needed:	Textbook; transparency masters 1 and 2; Behavior Modification Contracts
Goal Statement:	Participants will evaluate their own lifestyles through the Healthy Lifestyles Awareness Inventory and become familiar with the factors that have an impact on behavior modification.

EVALUATING YOUR LIFESTYLE

Time: 15 minutes

Instructor Notes

Purpose of Healthy Lifestyles

Primary Points:

- A healthy lifestyle is a combination of positive beliefs and practices.
- Our knowledge of healthy lifestyle practices will guide our actions and habits.
- Our personal beliefs and practices can increase or decrease risks of injury or sudden illness.
- Lifestyle changes we make now can prevent future injury and/or illness.

Healthy Lifestyles Awareness Inventory

Activity:

Having completed the Healthy Lifestyles Awareness Inventory as assigned, participants need to tally their scores, if they have not already done so. Have the participants record their scores on the Healthy Lifestyles Scorecard at the end of the inventory and turn it in to you. Tell participants that it is not necessary for them to put their names on the scorecard.

Textbook

Note: The purpose of having you receive all of the participants' scores is to tally the total class score for computing the class average. This activity will be completed again, at the end of the course, to determine if there has been an improvement in group behavior.

MAKING LIFESTYLE CHANGES

Time: 30 minutes

Modifying Behaviors

Primary Points:

Transparency Master 1

- Lifestyle changes require changes in behaviors.
- In order for changes in behavior to be successful—
  - An individual must want to change.
  - The desire to change must be accompanied by a change in attitude.
  - Changes in attitude must persist in order for long-term changes in behavior to succeed.

Strategies for Successful Behavior Changes

Transparency Master 2

- Evaluate pros and cons of current habits to determine what behaviors you want to change.
- Set short- and long-term goals.
- Use positive rewards for achieving both short- and long-term goals.
- Avoid situations that promote behaviors you are trying to change.
- Reinforce commitment to change by keeping your goal in front of you (post it on your refrigerator, mirror, and so on).
- Use the support of others.
- Get professional help if needed.

Developing a Behavior Modification Contract

Activity:

Textbook

Behavior Modification Contracts

1. Ask the participants to divide into small groups (three to four) to discuss the results of each participant's inventory for the purpose of identifying areas where improvement is possible.
2. Ask each participant to identify an area that he or she wants to improve. The group members will work as a team to help each other identify a measurable goal and objective(s) for improvement in that area during the course.
3. If you want to use it, have participants record their individual goals, objectives, and measures on a Behavior Modification Contract (Appendix N in this manual).
4. Ask participants how they feel about making a commitment like this. Ask them what roadblocks they anticipate to being successful.

Assignment:

Instruct participants that there is no reading assignment for the next lesson.

Lesson 3: THE CITIZEN RESPONDER

Class assignment prior to this lesson:	None
Length:	45 minutes
Needed:	Video; flip chart or chalkboard
Goal Statement:	The participants will become familiar with how the EMS system works and their roles as citizen responders in the EMS system.

DECIDING TO ACT

Instructor Notes

Time: 25 minutes

Video:

Tell participants that they are about to see a video showing an emergency situation. At the end, you will ask them to answer a few questions.

Show the video segment: *Barriers to Action* (05:00). Stop at end of this segment.

Note: If you do not have the video, you may use the scenario below to prepare participants for the activity that follows.

"A motorcycle with two riders weaves dangerously between parked cars in a crowded shopping center parking lot. As the cyclists dart between cars, they confront a moving truck. Both truck and cycle veer to avoid a head-on collision. The truck strikes several parked cars. The cycle strikes the side of the truck, throwing the riders to the ground.

Nearby, Jamie and Paul (two college students) hear the sound of crunching metal and blaring horns and decide to join the small group that has gathered. As they approach the scene, they are confronted with the sight of broken glass and metal, a cracked truck windshield, and a racing truck engine. A gas cap lies nearby, and they notice that gasoline has spilled from the cycle onto the roadway. One cyclist screams in pain as she sits holding her injured arms. The other cyclist lies motionless. Two people, wearing seat belts, are inside the truck. The driver appears to be shaken. Several onlookers turn away, apparently unable to confront the scene. Other bystanders continue to gather. As Jamie and Paul look around, no one seems to be willing to respond. They hesitate, wondering whether or not they should step forward to help. Would you?"

Activity:

1. Initiate a discussion about the difficulty of deciding to help, using the key questions below. Allow participants time to respond.
   - "How do you feel about what you just saw or experienced?"
   - "How many of you would respond to this emergency?"
   - "Those of you who wouldn't respond, why not?"
   - "Can anyone think of any other reasons that might discourage a person from responding?"

Note: Participants may or may not feel comfortable in responding. Be sensitive to each response. If a response seems odd to you or to the other participants, reinforce that some barriers to action are personal. What is a barrier to one person may not be to another. Carefully dispel myths that surface in the discussion.

2. Make a list of the participants' responses to the last question above.
   - When the list appears complete, explain that these are real barriers and can have an impact on the outcome for the victim.

Flip Chart/ Chalkboard

HELPING AT THE EMERGENCY SCENE

Time: 20 minutes

Activity:

1. Explain that providing help at an emergency scene does not always mean providing direct care for the victim(s). Ask—"In what other ways can help be given?"
2. Ask the participants to make a list of the steps they would take to help at this particular scene. Record the participants' responses.

Flip Chart/ Chalkboard

3. When the list appears complete, help the participants place the items in one of three categories:
   - Keeping the scene safe
   - Getting professional help
   - Giving care

   Then ask participants which category should be done first.

   Note: There is not necessarily a right or wrong answer as to which should be done first. Instead, participants need to realize that sometimes things are done simultaneously.

4. Ask participants to prioritize the steps for giving care. Guide their responses to help them focus on the injuries or conditions that are life-threatening.
5. Summarize the lesson by emphasizing that—
   - Deciding to help is not always an easy decision to make.
   - The presence of a crowd does not mean that someone is helping.
   - It is not always easy to determine how to help in an emergency.
   - There are many ways to help besides providing first aid care.
6. Explain to the participants that, in the next lesson, they will learn the Emergency Action Principles—four general steps to help them respond to any emergency situation.

Assignment: ◆ Read Chapters 1 and 3.

Lesson 4: RESPONDING TO EMERGENCIES

Class assignment prior to this lesson:	Read Chapters 1 and 3.
Length:	45 minutes
Needed:	Video; color transparencies 1 through 3; transparency masters 3 and 4
Goal Statement:	The participants will become familiar with the four Emergency Action Principles that provide a mental template for use in any emergency.

EMERGENCY ACTION PRINCIPLES

Instructor Notes

Time: 25 minutes

Primary Points:

- Briefly review the list of participant responses from the previous lesson regarding what steps to take to help in an emergency.

  Note: You will recall that the three general categories were scene safety, summoning professional help, and providing care.

- Summarize the participants' priorities by pointing out that priorities are generally classified into three categories. Explain that the emergency response generally needs to include four tasks:
  - Making sure the scene is safe
  - Summoning professional medical help
  - Caring for life-threatening emergencies until EMS personnel arrive
  - Caring for non-life-threatening emergencies

- The four Emergency Action Principles (EAPs) provide a mental template that will guide your actions in any emergency so that you can do these four tasks in the most appropriate manner:
  - Survey the scene.
  - Do a primary survey.
  - Call EMS personnel.
  - Do a secondary survey.

Color Transparency 1

Video:

Show the video segment: *Emergency Action Principles* (08:00).

Note: If you do not have the video, you may use the scenario below to prepare the participants for the activity that follows. You will notice that the first half of this scenario is the same as the one used in the previous lesson.

"A motorcycle with two riders weaves dangerously between parked cars in a crowded shopping center parking lot. As the cyclists dart between cars, they confront a moving truck. Both truck and cycle veer to avoid a head-on collision. The truck strikes several parked cars. The cycle strikes the side of the truck, throwing the riders to the ground.

Nearby, Jamie and Paul (two college students) hear the sound of crunching metal and blaring horns and decide to join the small group that has gathered. As they approach the scene they are confronted with the sight of broken glass and metal, a cracked truck windshield, and a racing truck engine. A gas cap lies nearby and they notice that gasoline has spilled from the cycle onto the roadway. One cyclist screams in pain as she sits holding her injured arms. The other cyclist lies motionless. Two people, wearing seat belts, are inside the truck. The driver appears to be shaken. Several onlookers turn away, apparently unable to confront the scene, while others gather. Jamie and Paul decide to step forward and help.

Jamie asks bystanders to help stop traffic. Paul asks the people in the truck to turn off the engine. The leaking gas from the motorcycle is not close to the cycle driver and passenger.

Jamie checks the cycle driver and determines he is unconscious but breathing. The two people in the car are conscious and talking to Paul. The other cyclist, still screaming, is attended to by another rescuer who helps control the bleeding from the cyclist's arm. Jamie, realizing that no one has called for an ambulance, now asks a bystander to do so.

Paul is able to do a secondary survey on the conscious, but confused, driver of the truck. The third rescuer also does a secondary survey on the injured, conscious cyclist."

Activity:

Use the list of key questions below to lead a discussion of Emergency Action Principles.

- What could have made this scene unsafe to approach?
- What steps were taken to ensure the scene's safety?
- Which responders performed a primary survey, and what were they specifically looking for?
- How was each primary survey performed?
- At what point did someone decide to call for help?
- What information should the caller give to the EMS dispatcher?
- Which responder(s) performed a secondary survey?
- Which responder(s) did not perform a secondary survey, and why not?
- What changes in the condition of the victim should a first aider look for while performing a secondary survey?

EMERGENCY MEDICAL SERVICES SYSTEM

Time: 5 minutes

Primary Points:

- The EMS system is made up of a chain of links that begins with recognizing an emergency and calling for help.
- The strength of the chain depends on the strength of each link. Each link is important in providing effective emergency response. If one fails, the system fails.

Color Transparency 2

Color Transparency 3

- Most people in the United States call a 9–1–1 emergency number. However, some areas still have a seven-digit local number.

Activity:

1. Ask participants to give examples of how an EMS system failure could occur.
2. Ask participants to identify the emergency number in their community (where they live, work, or go to school).

YOU ARE THE CITIZEN RESPONDER

Time: 15 minutes

Activity:

1. Read the following scenarios aloud to the class. Ask the participants to discuss briefly how to respond to each situation appropriately, using the EAPs to help guide their responses.

Scenario 1:
You see a car veer off the road, striking a utility pole. The pole splinters, dropping wires onto the vehicle. You decide to help. How would you respond?

Transparency Master 3

Scenario 2:
You arrive at your grandfather's home and find him lying motionless in the backyard. You hear a neighbor in the yard next door. You decide to help. How would you respond?

Scenario 3:
While jogging, you notice a bike rider fall as she rounds a corner on a rain-slick road. With her crumpled bike nearby, she is lying in the road moaning. You decide to help. How would you respond?

Transparency Master 4

Scenario 4:
During a softball game, a ball is hit between two players. Both converge on the ball. They collide, falling to the ground. One player is holding his arm, screaming in pain. The second player lies motion-

less. You decide to help. How would you respond?

2. Summarize by reinforcing that the four steps of the Emergency Action Principles will guide participants' actions in any emergency:
   - Survey the scene.
   - Do a primary survey.
   - Call EMS.
   - Do a secondary survey.

Color Transparency 1

Assignment:

◆ Read Chapter 2.

Lesson 5: BODY SYSTEMS

Class assignment prior to this lesson:	Read Chapter 2.
Length:	45 minutes
Needed:	Video; color transparencies 4 through 14
Goal Statement:	The participants will become familiar with the major structures and primary functions of each body system and gain an understanding of how body systems work together. They will also become familiar with the signals that may indicate a problem with one or more systems when an injury or illness occurs.

UNDERSTANDING THE HUMAN BODY

Instructor Notes

Time: 30 minutes

Primary Points:

- Review the Emergency Action Principles.
- Explain that information about body systems will help participants to better understand the reasons for the primary and secondary survey steps of the EAPs.
- Knowledge of how body systems normally function will help the citizen responder understand what happens when body systems fail.

Video:

Show the video segment: *Understanding the Human Body* (11:00).

Note: If you choose not to show this video segment, develop a brief lecture on the information in Chapter 2. Include each of the body systems, the major structures and functions, and what happens when the body systems fail. Give examples of how body systems work together and how other body systems are affected when one body system fails.

Activity:

Using the transparencies, ask the participants to identify the major body systems, their structures, and functions. Use the questions below to guide the participants' responses for each body system.

Color Transparencies 4 through 14

- What are the major structures of this system?
- What is this system's primary function?
- How can you recognize that it is working properly?
- What are some indications that it is not working properly?

INTERRELATIONSHIPS AMONG BODY SYSTEMS

Time: 15 minutes

Activity:

You may use the same transparencies and the following examples to reinforce the interrelationships among the body systems by giving examples of problems that may arise from injuries or sudden illnesses.

Color Transparencies 4 through 14

Nervous system:
A serious head injury. A head injury may affect the respiratory system, causing breathing to stop.

Skeletal system:
A broken bone in the arm. An injury to a bone can sever a blood vessel or pinch a nerve, impairing the flow of blood or causing loss of feeling below the injury site.

Circulatory system:
Heart attack. A heart attack impairs the circulatory system, preventing delivery of oxygen-rich blood to vital organs such as the brain.

Respiratory system:
Choking. A blockage in the airway does not permit air to reach the lungs, preventing oxygen from being circulated to the vital organs. As a result, the heart will stop and brain cells will die.

Assignment:

- Review key terms and the major body systems (Table 2–1, page 22).
- Review Chapter 3 skill sheet: Primary Survey (pages 64 and 65).

Lesson 6: PRIMARY/SECONDARY SURVEY I

Class assignment prior to this lesson:	Review key terms and major body systems (Table 2–1, page 22). Review Chapter 3 skill sheet: Primary Survey (pages 64 and 65).
Length:	45 minutes
Needed:	Video; transparency master 5; Participant Progress Log; skill sheet; blankets or mats
Goal Statement:	The participants will become familiar with how to perform a primary survey on an unconscious victim.

PERFORMING A PRIMARY SURVEY

Instructor Notes

Time: 10 minutes

Video:

Show the video segment: *Primary and Secondary Survey* (04:00). Stop the video at first pause point when the primary survey segment is completed.

Note: If you do not have the video, you may briefly discuss the following primary points.

Primary Points:

Transparency Master 5

- During the primary survey, check and care for life-threatening conditions.
- When doing a primary survey, check for consciousness. Then check the ABCs.
- The primary survey should be done in the position in which you find the victim. If you cannot check the ABCs or if the victim is not breathing, position the victim on the back.
- A victim who can speak, cough, or cry is conscious, has an open airway, is breathing, and has a pulse.

SKILL PRACTICE: PRIMARY SURVEY

Time: 35 minutes

Position the Victim

Activity:

Skill Sheet

Participant Progress Log

1. Ask the participants to take their skill sheets with them to the practice area.
2. Assign partners or ask participants to find partners.

3. Tell participants that they will practice positioning a victim, using their partner to simulate a facedown, unconscious victim.
4. Guide the participants as they practice, giving help when appropriate or when requested.
5. After participants have practiced the skills to the point at which they feel comfortable in their ability to perform them, have the participants change places. Repeat the practice. Check participants' skills as you watch them practice.

Blankets or Mats

Primary Survey

Activity:

1. Tell the participants that they will practice the primary survey on their partner.
2. Instruct the participants to find their own carotid pulse. Ask them to find their partner's carotid pulse.
3. Have participants practice performing a primary survey on an unconscious, breathing person.

   Note: Participants will not do a pulse check, since this victim is breathing. However, they should still check for severe bleeding.

4. Have participants practice performing a primary survey on an unconscious, **nonbreathing** person.

   Note: Participants will need to do a pulse check once they have checked and been told that the person is not breathing. In addition, the participants should identify or simulate two initial rescue breaths.

5. Guide the participants through the skill. Watch participants as they practice, giving help when appropriate or when requested.
6. After participants have practiced the skills to the point at which they feel comfortable in their ability to perform

Skill Sheet

Participant Progress Log

Blankets or Mats

them, have the participants change places. Repeat the practice. Check participants' skills as you watch them practice.

7. Answer any questions that participants may have.

Assignment:

- Review Chapter 3 skill sheet: Secondary Survey (pages 66 through 69).

Lesson 7: PRIMARY/SECONDARY SURVEY II

Class assignment prior to this lesson:	Review Chapter 3 skill sheet: Secondary Survey (pages 66 through 69).
Length:	45 minutes
Needed:	Video; transparency master 6; Participant Progress Log; skill sheet; blankets or mats
Goal Statement:	The participants will become familiar with how to perform a secondary survey and when a secondary survey is appropriate.

PERFORMING A SECONDARY SURVEY

Instructor Notes

Time: 10 minutes

Video:

Show the second part of the video segment: *Primary and Secondary Survey* (07:00). Stop the video at the pause point.

Note: If you do not have the video, you may briefly discuss the following primary points.

Primary Points:

- ◆ When doing a primary survey, check for consciousness. Then check the ABCs.
- ◆ A victim who can speak, cough, or cry is conscious, has an open airway, is breathing, and has a pulse.
- ◆ The secondary survey is only done when no life-threatening emergencies are found in the primary survey.
- ◆ The secondary survey has three basic steps:
  - Interview the victim and bystanders to attempt to get information about the injury/illness.
  - Check the victim's vital signs.
  - Do a head-to-toe examination.
- ◆ The interview provides information that may be helpful to arriving EMS personnel.
- ◆ The focus on checking vital signs is to look for any changes in pulse, breathing, or skin.
- ◆ When doing a head-to-toe examination, remember not to have the victim move any painful areas.

Transparency Master 6

SKILL PRACTICE: SECONDARY SURVEY

Time: 35 minutes

Secondary Survey

Activity:

1. Ask participants to take their skill sheets with them to the practice area.
2. Assign partners or ask participants to find partners.
3. Tell participants that they will practice doing a secondary survey on each other.
4. Instruct the participants in how to find their own radial pulse. Ask them to find their partner's radial pulse.
5. Guide the participants through the skill of doing a secondary survey on a conscious injured person. Watch participants as they practice, giving help when appropriate or when requested.

   Note: To help focus the victim's responses during the interview portion of the secondary survey, create a simple scenario before you begin. For example, tell the victims that they have fallen and have injured their right knee.
6. After participants have practiced the skills to the point at which they feel comfortable in their ability to perform them, have the participants change places. Repeat the practice. Check participants' skills as you watch them practice.
7. Repeat the exercise, giving participants a simple scenario in which someone has suddenly become ill.
8. Inform participants that the next lesson focuses on what to do if someone is having difficulty breathing or is not breathing.

Skill Sheet

Participant Progress Log

Blankets or Mats

Assignment:

- Read Chapter 4.

Lesson 8: RESPIRATORY EMERGENCIES I

Class assignment prior to this lesson: Read Chapter 4.

Length: 45 minutes

Needed: Color transparencies 5 through 7; transparency masters 7 through 9; flip chart or chalkboard

Goal Statement: Using the primary survey, the participants will become familiar with the signals that indicate respiratory distress and make decisions regarding care for a person who is having difficulty breathing.

RESPIRATORY SYSTEM REVIEW

Instructor Notes

Time: 10 minutes

Primary Points:

Color Transparencies 5 through 7

- The respiratory system consists of the upper and lower airway and the lungs.
- The primary systems that work together for breathing to occur are the respiratory, circulatory, and nervous systems.
- The diaphragm and chest muscles contract and relax during inhalation and exhalation.
- Breathing emergencies are detected during the primary survey.
- Breathing emergencies include respiratory distress and respiratory arrest.
- By recognizing respiratory distress and taking immediate action, you may prevent respiratory arrest.

RECOGNIZING BREATHING EMERGENCIES

Time: 15 minutes

Causes of Breathing Emergencies

Activity:

Flip Chart/ Chalkboard

- Ask the participants to identify causes of breathing emergencies. Record the responses.

Note: Prompt the participants as necessary. Participant responses should include: choking; heart attack or heart disease; lung disease, asthma, injury to the chest or lungs; allergic reactions to food or drugs, insect bites or stings; drowning or near-drowning; electrocution; poisoning; shock.

Signals of Respiratory Distress

Activity:

- Ask the participants to identify signals of respiratory distress. Record the responses.

  Note: Participants' responses should include: anxiety; gasping for air; unusually fast or slow breathing; unusually shallow or deep breathing; unusually noisy breathing; painful breathing; dizziness; feeling short of breath; tingling in the hands or feet; moist, pale, bluish, or flushed skin.

Flip Chart/ Chalkboard

- Three common causes of respiratory distress are asthma, hyperventilation, and anaphylactic shock.

Transparency Master 7

COMMON TYPES OF RESPIRATORY DISTRESS

Time: 10 minutes

Asthma

Transparency Master 8

Primary Points:

- It is a condition that narrows the air passages and makes breathing difficult.
- It is more common in children than adults.
- It is commonly triggered by allergic reactions to pollen, food, a drug, or an insect sting, or can be caused by emotional stress or physical activity.
- Asthma attacks are usually controlled by medication.
- The characteristic signal of asthma is wheezing when exhaling.

Hyperventilation

Primary Points:

- It is a condition that occurs when someone breathes faster than normal.
- Rapid breathing upsets the body's balance of oxygen and carbon dioxide.

- It is often the result of fear or anxiety but can be caused by injuries to the head, severe bleeding, or some illnesses.
- It can also be triggered by asthma or exercise.
- The characteristic signal of hyperventilation is shallow, rapid breathing. Victims may also say that they feel dizzy or that their fingers and toes feel numb or tingly.

Anaphylactic Shock
(Also known as anaphylaxis)

Primary Points:

- It is a condition that results in swelling of the air passages, restricting breathing.
- It is usually caused by a severe allergic reaction to food, insect stings, or a medication such as penicillin.
- Signals include skin rash; tightness in the chest and throat; swelling of the face, neck, and tongue.

FIRST AID FOR RESPIRATORY DISTRESS

Time: 10 minutes

Primary Points:

- Respiratory distress may signal the beginning of a life-threatening condition.
- Respiratory distress may lead to respiratory arrest if not cared for immediately.
- Signals of different kinds of respiratory distress are often similar. You do not need to know the specific cause to provide care.
- Follow the EAPs to provide general care.
- Specifically, position a person in respiratory distress in a sitting position. This often helps alleviate some of the difficulty.
- If a room is hot or stuffy, open a window. Reducing heat and humidity often helps.

Transparency Master 9

Assignment:

- Review Chapter 4, and the skill sheet: Rescue Breathing for an Adult (pages 99 through 101).
- Read "Health Precautions and Guidelines for First Aid Training" and "Guidelines to Follow During Training" in the textbook (pages xx and xxi).

Note: Remind participants to dress comfortably for the next class's skill practice and to wash hands before coming into the classroom.

Lesson 9: RESPIRATORY EMERGENCIES II

Class assignment prior to this lesson: Review Chapter 4, skill sheet: Rescue Breathing for an Adult (pages 99 through 101). Read "Health Precautions and Guidelines for First Aid Training" and "Guidelines to Follow During Training" in the textbook (pages xx and xxi).

Length: 45 minutes

Needed: Textbook; video; transparency master 10; Participant Progress Log; skill sheet; decontamination supplies; manikins; blankets or mats

Goal Statement: Using the primary survey, the participants will become familiar with the signals of respiratory arrest and how to provide care for a person who is not breathing.

RESPIRATORY ARREST

Time: 5 minutes

Primary Points:

- Respiratory arrest is a life-threatening condition in which breathing stops.
- It is commonly caused by illness, injury, or choking.
- Respiratory distress, if uncared for, can lead to respiratory arrest.
- In respiratory arrest, body systems will progressively fail due to a lack of oxygen-rich blood circulating to the cells.
- Rescue breathing is a way of supplying oxygen to a nonbreathing person by breathing air into the lungs.
- Rescue breathing works because the air you exhale contains more than enough oxygen to keep the victim alive.
- Rescue breathing is the first aid you provide someone who is not breathing but has a pulse.
- You will determine if a victim needs rescue breathing during the primary survey.

Instructor Notes

Transparency Master 10

FIRST AID FOR RESPIRATORY ARREST

Time: 10 minutes

Video:

Show the video segment: *The Primary Survey: Rescue Breathing* (05:30). Stop the video at the pause point.

Note: If you choose not to show this video segment, provide a demonstration of rescue breathing, beginning with the primary survey. Ensure that all participants can see the demonstration.

Primary Points:

- When doing a primary survey, start by checking consciousness. Then check the ABCs.
- Sometimes the tongue is blocking the airway. The head-tilt/chin-lift technique opens the airway by moving the tongue away from the back of the throat.
- Open the airway to check for breathing.
- If the victim is not breathing but has a pulse, do rescue breathing.
- Give one full breath every five seconds.
- Blow in slowly until the chest rises.
- Give rescue breathing for one minute, about 12 breaths, and then recheck pulse.

SKILL PRACTICE: RESCUE BREATHING

Time: 20 minutes

Activity:

1. Briefly review the "Health Precautions for First Aid Training" and "Guidelines to Follow During Training." Refer the participants to pages xx and xxi in their textbook.
2. Tell the participants that they will practice rescue breathing on a manikin.
3. Demonstrate how to properly clean the manikin following use. Keep the manikin on its back at all times in order to keep the face clean.

Textbook

4. Move the participants into the practice area.
5. Assign partners or ask participants to find partners.
6. Guide the participants through the skill. Watch participants as they practice, giving help when appropriate, or when requested.

Skill Sheet

Decontamination Supplies

Manikins

Blankets or Mats

Note: Remember, the participants have already learned the basic mechanics of conducting the primary survey in previous lessons. Their attention should focus on the recognition of a nonbreathing victim, giving rescue breaths, and then putting it all together.

7. After participants have practiced the skills to the point at which they feel comfortable in their ability to perform them, have the participants change places. Repeat the practice. Check participants' skills as you watch them practice.

Participant Progress Log

8. Answer any questions that the participants may have.

PRIMARY SURVEY REVIEW

Time: 10 minutes

Video: Show the video segment: *Primary Survey: Putting It All Together* (09:00). Stop the video at the pause point.

Note: If you do not have the video, you may briefly review the primary survey.

Assignment:

- Review Chapter 4 skill sheets: Complete Airway Obstruction (unconscious adult) and Complete Airway Obstruction (conscious adult), pages 102 through 107.

Note: Remind participants to dress comfortably for skill practice and to wash their hands before coming into the classroom.

Lesson 10: RESPIRATORY EMERGENCIES III

Class assignment prior to this lesson: Review Chapter 4 skill sheets: Complete Airway Obstruction (unconscious adult) and Complete Airway Obstruction (conscious adult), pages 102 through 107.

Length: 45 minutes

Needed: Video; transparency master 11; Participant Progress Log; skill sheet; decontamination supplies; manikins; blankets or mats

Goal Statement: Using the primary survey, the participants will become familiar with the signals of a choking emergency and make decisions regarding care for a person who is choking.

AIRWAY OBSTRUCTION

Time: 5 minutes

Instructor Notes

Transparency Master 11

Primary Points:

- Airway obstruction is the most common respiratory emergency.
- There are two types of airway obstruction—anatomical and mechanical.
- An obstruction is called anatomical if the airway is blocked by an anatomic structure such as the tongue or swollen tissues of the mouth and throat.
- The most common cause of obstruction in an unconscious person is the tongue, which drops to the back of the throat and blocks the airway.
- An obstruction is called mechanical if the airway is blocked by a foreign object, such as a piece of food, a small toy, or fluids such as vomit, blood, mucus, or saliva. Someone with a mechanical obstruction is said to be choking.
- A person who is choking may have either a complete or partial airway obstruction.
- A person with a partial airway obstruction can still move air to and from the lungs, which enables him or her to be able to cough in an attempt to dislodge the object.
- A person with a complete airway obstruction is unable to speak, breathe, or cough.

FIRST AID FOR AIRWAY OBSTRUCTION

Time: 10 minutes

Video:

Show the video segment: *The Primary Survey/Obstructed Airway* (08:00). Stop the video at the pause point.

Note: If you do not have the video you may briefly discuss the following primary points.

Primary Points:

- Review with participants that the tongue is the most common cause of obstructed airway in an unconscious victim. You must position the victim so that the tongue does not block the airway.
- The head-tilt/chin-lift technique opens the airway by moving the tongue from the back of the throat.
- If you determine during the primary survey that the airway is blocked by a foreign object, attempt to remove it by giving abdominal thrusts.

SKILL PRACTICE: OBSTRUCTED AIRWAY

Time: 30 minutes

Complete Airway Obstruction (unconscious adult)

Activity:

1. Move the participants into the practice area.
2. Assign partners or ask participants to find partners.
3. Tell the participants that they will practice first aid on a manikin for an unconscious victim whose airway is obstructed.
4. Guide the participants through the skill. Watch the participants as they practice, giving help when appropriate or when requested.
5. After participants have practiced the skills to the point at which they feel comfortable in their ability to perform them, have the participants change places. Repeat the practice. Check participants' skills as you watch them practice.

Skill Sheet

Decontamination Supplies

Manikins

Blankets or Mats

Participant Progress Log

Complete Airway Obstruction (conscious adult)

1. Tell the participants that they will practice first aid for a conscious victim whose airway is obstructed on their partner, but they **will not** give actual abdominal thrusts.
2. Have participants stand in a line or semicircle with their partners behind them.
3. Guide the participants through the skill. Watch the participants as they practice, giving them help when appropriate or when needed.
4. After participants have practiced the skills to the point at which they feel comfortable in their ability to perform them, have the participants change places. Repeat the practice. Check participants' skills as you watch them practice.
5. Answer any questions that the participants may have.

Participant Progress Log

Assignment:

- Read Chapter 5.
- Bring the Healthy Lifestyles Awareness Inventory to the next class.

Lesson 11: CARDIAC EMERGENCIES I

Class assignment prior to this lesson:	Read Chapter 5. Bring the Healthy Lifestyles Inventory Awareness to class.
Length:	45 minutes
Needed:	Video; color transparencies 8, 15 through 17; transparency masters 12 and 13; flip chart or chalkboard
Goal Statement:	The participants will become familiar with the signals of a heart attack and how to care for a victim who experiences these signals. The participants will also become aware of how to identify and reduce risk factors for cardiovascular disease that could lead to a heart attack.

CARDIOVASCULAR SYSTEM REVIEW

Time: 5 minutes

Instructor Notes

Primary Points:

- The circulatory system consists of the heart, blood, and blood vessels.
- The circulatory system works with the respiratory system to carry oxygen to every cell in the body.
- The heart is a muscular organ located behind the breastbone.
- The heart pumps blood throughout the body through arteries and veins.
- Arteries carry oxygen-rich blood to the cells, and veins carry oxygen-poor blood from the cells to the lungs.
- The pumping action of the heart is called a contraction.
- Contractions are controlled by the heart's electrical system, which makes the heart beat regularly.
- You can feel the heart's contractions in the arteries that are close to the skin (such as in the neck or wrist).
- The beat you feel with each contraction is called the pulse.

Color Transparencies 8 and 15

RECOGNIZING A HEART ATTACK

Time: 25 minutes

Video: Show the video segment: *Recognizing a Heart Attack* (11:30). Stop the video at the next pause point.

Note: If you do not have the video, use the entire 25 minutes for discussion.

Activity:

Flip Chart/ Chalkboard

1. Initiate a discussion by asking the participants if they have ever observed a victim who was showing signals of a heart attack. Ask the participants to explain what specific signals they saw, what care was given, and how bystanders responded. Allow participants time to respond.
   - If none of the participants have an experience to share, use the video that they just saw to get responses or describe an experience you have witnessed or heard about.
2. Compare participants' experiences of signals to those on the video or that you describe. Make a list of the signals, such as the primary one—chest pain. Others should include—trouble breathing, nausea or vomiting, sweating, ill appearance or feeling.

Specific Signals of Heart Attack

Primary Points:

Color Transparencies 16 and 17

- Explain that heart attacks are commonly caused by a narrowing of, or blockage in, the arteries that supply the heart muscle.
- This results in insufficient blood flow and, therefore, insufficient oxygen.
- This results in the most prominent signal of heart attack—persistent chest pain.
- This pain is usually felt in the center of the chest behind the sternum but may radiate into the neck, shoulder, or arms.
- Victims describe it as uncomfortable pressure, squeezing, or tightness.
- The pain is constant and not relieved by rest or medication.

- Any severe chest pain, pain lasting longer than 10 minutes, or pain accompanied by other signals should receive immediate medical attention.

Caring for a Heart Attack

Primary Points:

- Have the person stop all physical activity and rest.
- Position the person so that he or she can rest comfortably. This is usually a sitting position.
- Call EMS personnel immediately.
- Keep a calm reassuring manner.
- Monitor vital signs, looking for changes in appearance or behavior.

Transparency Master 12

RISK FACTORS FOR CARDIOVASCULAR DISEASE

Time: 15 minutes

Reviewing Healthy Lifestyles Awareness Inventory

Activity:

1. Ask the participants to identify the risk factors of cardiovascular disease (CVD). Record their responses.
2. Ask the participants to review their own Healthy Lifestyles Awareness Inventory to determine how many of these risk factors apply to them.
3. Ask the participants to indicate by a show of hands, how many have no risk factors for CVD...how many have one risk factor for CVD...how many have two or more risk factors? Explain that your risks don't just **add**, they **multiply**.
4. Of those who have one or more risk factors, ask how many of them can eliminate at least one risk by making lifestyle changes now.
5. Ask the participants to give examples of lifestyle changes that will reduce the risk of CVD.
6. Ask if any participants have as a goal on the Behavior Modification Contract to make changes that will reduce their own risk of CVD.

Flip Chart/ Chalkboard

Transparency Master 13

7. Explain the importance of reducing CVD **now** because it develops gradually, over many years. Therefore, leading a healthier lifestyle now is important for their future health.

Assignment:

- Review Chapter 5 skill sheet: CPR for an Adult (pages 131 to 135).

Note: Remind participants to dress comfortably for skill practice and to wash hands before coming into the classroom.

Lesson 12: CARDIAC EMERGENCIES II

Class assignment prior to this lesson: Review Chapter 5 skill sheet: CPR for an Adult (pages 131 through 135).

Length: 45 minutes

Needed: Video; color transparencies 16 through 18; transparency masters 12 and 14; skill sheet; decontamination supplies; manikins; blankets or mats

Goal Statement: Using the primary survey, the participants will become familiar with how to recognize the signals of cardiac arrest and make decisions regarding care of a victim of a cardiac emergency.

HEART ATTACK

Time: 5 minutes

Instructor Notes

Review Signals of a Heart Attack

Primary Points:

- Heart attacks are commonly caused by a narrowing of, or blockage in, the arteries that supply the heart muscle.
- The most prominent signal of a heart attack is persistent chest pain.
- Heart attack pain is commonly felt in the center of the chest behind the sternum.
- Victims often describe it as an uncomfortable pressure, squeezing, tightness, aching, constricting, or heavy sensation in the chest. It may spread to the shoulder, arm, neck, or jaw.
- The pain is constant and usually not relieved by resting, changing positions, or taking medication.
- Any severe chest pain, chest pain that lasts longer than 10 minutes, or chest pain that is accompanied by other signals, should receive emergency medical care immediately.
- Other signals of heart attack include looking and feeling ill, nausea and vomiting, sweating, and breathing difficulty.

Color Transparencies 16 and 17

Review Caring for a Heart Attack

Primary Points:

- Have a person experiencing persistent chest pain rest comfortably. A sitting position will usually enable the person to breathe more easily.
- Call EMS personnel immediately.
- Keep a calm and reassuring manner. Continue to monitor the vital signs, looking for any changes in appearance or behavior. Be prepared to give CPR.

Transparency Master 12

CARDIAC ARREST

Time: 10 minutes

Primary Points:

- Cardiac arrest occurs when the heart stops beating or beats too irregularly or too weakly to circulate blood effectively.
- Besides CVD, the number one cause of cardiac arrest, other causes include: drowning, suffocation, electrocution, poisoning, respiratory arrest, or injuries causing severe blood loss.
- A victim in cardiac arrest is unconscious, not breathing, and without a pulse.
- Not all cardiac arrest victims will show signals of a heart attack before the arrest. This is called sudden death.
- Care for cardiac arrest is CPR given by a bystander followed quickly by advanced cardiac life support by trained medical professionals.

Transparency Master 14

Video:

Show the video segment: *The Primary Survey: CPR* (07:30). Stop the video at the pause point.

Note: If you choose not to use the video, provide a demonstration of CPR, starting with the primary survey. Make sure that all of the participants are able to see the demonstration.

Primary Points:

- Signals of cardiac arrest will be found during the primary survey.
- Do not rush the breathing and pulse checks. Take about 5 seconds for the breathing check and about 10 seconds for the pulse check.
- Locate the correct compression position each time before giving compressions. Ask the participants to find the notch on themselves where the ribs and sternum meet.
- Explain that chest compressions should be done with the heel of the hand and to press evenly while counting.

Color Transparency 18

SKILL PRACTICE: CPR—CHEST COMPRESSIONS ONLY

Time: 30 minutes

Activity:

1. Move the participants into the practice area.
2. Assign partners or ask participants to find partners.
3. Using manikins, have participants go through the steps of the primary survey up to the pulse check. At this point, guide participants in finding proper compression position and giving compressions. Watch the participants as they practice, giving help when appropriate or when requested.
4. After participants have practiced the skills to the point at which they feel comfortable in their ability to perform them, have the participants change places. Repeat the practice. Check participants' skills as you watch them.
5. Answer any questions that participants may have.

Skill Sheets

Decontamination Supplies

Blankets or Mats

Manikins

Assignment:

- Review Chapter 5 skill sheet: CPR for an Adult (pages 131 through 135).

Lesson 13: CARDIAC EMERGENCIES III

Class assignment prior to this lesson: Review Chapter 5 skill sheet: CPR for an Adult (pages 131 through 135).

Length: 45 minutes

Needed: Participant Progress Log; skill sheet; decontamination supplies; manikins; blankets or mats

Goal Statement: Participants will become familiar with the technique of CPR.

SKILL PRACTICE: CPR

Time: 45 minutes

Activity:

1. Move the participants into the practice area.
2. Assign partners or ask participants to find partners.
3. Review locating proper hand position and giving compressions.
4. When participants have mastered these techniques, add giving rescue breaths alternately with sets of compressions.
5. Instruct the participants to practice CPR, beginning with the primary survey. Watch participants as they practice, giving help when appropriate or when requested.
6. After participants have practiced the skill to the point at which they feel comfortable in their ability to perform it, have them change places. Repeat the practice. Check participants' skills as you watch them practice.
7. Answer any questions that participants may have.

Assignment:

- Read Chapters 6 and 7.

Instructor Notes

Skill Sheets

Decontamination Supplies

Manikins

Blankets or Mats

Participant Progress Log

Lesson 14: BLEEDING AND SHOCK

Class assignment prior to this lesson: Read Chapters 6 and 7.

Length: 45 minutes

Needed: Video; color transparencies 19 and 20; transparency masters 15 through 21; gauze pads; roller bandages.

Goal Statement: The participants will become familiar with the conditions that can result in shock, and describe the signals and care for shock. They will also become familiar with the primary signals of internal bleeding and life-threatening bleeding and describe how to control each.

REVIEW OF THE CIRCULATORY SYSTEM

Time: 5 minutes

Instructor Notes

Primary Points:

- The circulatory system consists of the heart, blood, and blood vessels.

  Transparency Master 15

- Escape of blood from arteries, veins, or capillaries is called bleeding.
- Blood is made up of liquid (plasma) and solid components (white and red blood cells and platelets).
- Blood has three major functions:

  Transparency Master 16

  - Protects against disease
  - Maintains constant body temperature
  - Transports oxygen, nutrients, and wastes
- Three major types of blood vessels are arteries, capillaries, and veins.
- Blood in the arteries travels faster and under greater pressure than blood in capillaries or veins.
- Blood in the arteries pulses with each contraction of the heart; blood in the veins flows more slowly and evenly.
- Bleeding is either internal or external. External bleeding is generally obvious.
- Uncontrolled bleeding, whether internal or external, is a life-threatening emergency.

- When bleeding occurs, blood volume is affected. Significant loss in blood volume will be life-threatening. Therefore, severe bleeding should be controlled immediately.

EXTERNAL BLEEDING

Time: 15 minutes

Signals of External Bleeding

Primary Points:

Transparency Master 17

- Each type of blood vessel bleeds differently because blood pressure within the vessels varies.
- Arterial bleeding is often rapid and profuse. Because it is under more pressure, it spurts from the wound. It is harder to control than other types of bleeding.
- Venous blood is under less pressure and flows from the wound at a steady rate.
- Capillary bleeding is under low pressure and "oozes" from the wound.

Controlling External Bleeding

Primary Points:

Transparency Master 18

Gauze Pads

- External bleeding is usually easy to control.
- Placing a clean object, such as a gauze pad, on a wound will minimize infection.
- Applying direct pressure with the hand will stop most bleeding, allowing clots to form. (By allowing the victim to apply the pressure, disease transmission is minimized.)
- Elevating the injured area slows flow of blood and helps clotting.

Roller Bandages

- Pressure on a wound can be maintained by snugly applying a bandage—a pressure bandage.
- If bleeding cannot be controlled, arteries can be compressed against the underlying bone at specific sites on the body, called pressure points, to help stop otherwise uncontrollable bleeding.

- Brachial (arms) and femoral (legs) arteries can be used to control bleeding in the extremities.
- Summon EMS personnel if bleeding cannot be controlled or if pressure points must be used to control it.

Video:

Show the video segment: *Severe Bleeding* (03:00). Stop the the video at the pause point.

Note: If you do not choose to use the video, briefly discuss situations in which participants may need to control severe bleeding while dealing with other life-threatening emergencies.

INTERNAL BLEEDING

Time: 5 minutes

Signals of Internal Bleeding

Primary Points:

- Internal bleeding is the escape of blood from arteries, veins, or capillaries into spaces within the body.
- Internal bleeding is not directly visible, and it may take time for signals to appear.
- Suspect internal bleeding in any serious injury.
- Signals include—
  - Discoloration of the skin (bruising).
  - Tissues that are tender, swollen, or hard—such as those in the abdomen.
  - Anxiety or restlessness.
  - Rapid breathing.
  - Skin that feels cool or moist or looks pale or bluish.
  - Nausea and vomiting.
  - Excessive thirst.
  - Declining level of consciousness.

Color Transparency 19

Transparency Master 19

Controlling Internal Bleeding

Primary Points:

- Care depends on severity and site.
- If there is minor internal bleeding, such as bruising, apply ice to the injured area to reduce pain and swelling.
- If you suspect that internal bleeding is likely because of the seriousness of an injury, call EMS immediately; shock may result, and there is little you can do.

SHOCK

Time: 10 minutes

Signals of Shock

Primary Points:

Color Transparency 20

- Shock is a life-threatening condition in which the circulatory system fails to circulate oxygen-rich blood to all parts of the body.
- It is the inevitable result of any serious injury or illness.
- When vital organs are affected, it triggers a series of responses that produce specific signals, collectively known as shock.
- These signals are a result of the body's attempt to maintain adequate blood flow to vital organs, preventing their failure. The signals of shock are—
  - Restlessness or irritability. This is the earliest indicator of shock and is due to insufficient oxygen in the brain.
  - Rapid and weak pulse.
  - Rapid breathing.
  - Pale or bluish, cool, moist skin.
  - Excessive thirst.
  - Nausea and vomiting.
  - Drowsiness or loss of consciousness.
- Signals of shock may be present immediately, become evident during the secondary survey, or appear later.

Caring for Shock

Primary Points:

- Follow the EAPs—Do a primary survey checking ABCs. If there are no life-threatening conditions, do a secondary survey.
- Provide general care. Be proactive, not reactive. Do not wait for signals of shock to appear before providing care.
  - Do no further harm.
  - Monitor ABCs.
  - Help the victim rest comfortably. Unless the victim is having great difficulty breathing, he or she may be most comfortable lying down.
  - Help the victim to maintain normal body temperature.
  - Reassure the victim.
  - Provide care for specific conditions.
- Specifically—
  - Control external bleeding as soon as possible.
  - Elevate the legs unless you suspect head or spine injuries or possible broken bones involving hips or legs.
  - Give nothing to eat or drink.
  - Call EMS personnel immediately.

Transparency Master 20

YOU ARE THE CITIZEN RESPONDER

Time: 10 minutes

Activity:

1. Read the following scenario aloud to the class.
2. Initiate a discussion using the key questions that follow the scenario.

Note: As the scenario unfolds, additional information is given to encourage the participants to think how they could respond.

Scenario
Conscious Person, Breathing, With Severe Bleeding

Transparency Master 21

You are hiking with a friend on a marked trail in a local park. You both decide to stray from this path in search of more challenging terrain. Your friend loses his footing on loose rocks and falls approximately 15 feet down the rocky incline. When you reach him, you notice that he is bleeding badly from a deep wound on the lower leg.

- How would you provide care?

In attempting to control bleeding, you raise your friend's leg. He cries out in pain.

- How do you react?
- Does your care change?

After several minutes have passed, you notice that your friend appears pale and is sweating. He tells you he is feeling a little dizzy and nauseated. He asks for water from your canteen.

- How do you respond?

Note: Participant should begin by making sure the scene is safe, followed by a primary survey. With the awareness that the person is breathing, the participant knows there is a pulse and should scan the body for severe bleeding. Seeing that the lower leg is bleeding heavily, the participant should take steps to control the bleeding.

If raising the leg to elevate the wound above the level of the heart causes pain, participant should lower the leg to the ground and minimize any further movement. Participant should shout for help in an effort to attract any nearby hikers.

The injured person is beginning to show signals of shock. The participant should refuse the victim water, and summon emergency personnel immediately. This may mean leaving his or her friend, or sending any passerby who responded to the shouts for help.

3. Answer any questions that participants may have.

Assignment:

- Review Chapters 1 through 7 and complete any unanswered Study Questions.

Lesson 15: PUTTING IT ALL TOGETHER I

Class assignment prior to this lesson:	Review Chapters 1 through 7. Complete unanswered Study Questions.
Length:	45 minutes
Needed:	Color transparency 1; transparency masters 22 through 26; self-assessment exercise 1; blankets or mats; manikins (optional); decontamination supplies
Goal Statement:	Given a series of scenarios involving life-threatening and non-life-threatening situations, participants will be able to make appropriate decisions for care and demonstrate proper first aid techniques.

YOU ARE THE CITIZEN RESPONDER

Time: 45 minutes

Activity:

1. Divide the participants into small groups. Give each group one of the "Putting It All Together" scenarios. (See pages 95 through 96 in this manual.)
2. Tell the participants they will be given 10 minutes to formulate how best to respond to the emergency situation they have been given.
3. Remind the participants that they should use the Emergency Action Principles to guide their responses.
4. After 10 minutes, ask each group to role-play their scenario to the rest of the class. Each scenario should take about 10 minutes.

   Note: It is unlikely that all groups will be able to role-play their scenarios during this class. Time has been allowed for remaining groups in the next lesson.

5. One at a time, use the transparencies, or have participants read their scenario aloud to the class and role-play their response to their emergency. Tell the participants that they should demonstrate any previously-learned skill that would be required as an effective response.

Instructor Notes

Blankets or Mats

Manikins (optional)

Decontamination Supplies

Color Transparency 1

They may choose to use either a manikin or a member of the group as the victim at any time during the role play. Each group should discuss their actions while giving care. They should also be able to answer questions the instructor or other participants may have.

Note: If the group feels it is necessary to use a skill they have not learned, they may simply explain their actions and will not be required to demonstrate that skill (for example, actual bandaging procedures).

6. After a group has role-played their scenario, initiate a discussion by asking the class to evaluate the group's response, using the questions below.

   The Plan of Action

   - Did the group's plan follow the Emergency Action Principles?
     - Survey the scene
     - Primary survey
     - Call EMS
     - Secondary survey
   - Did the plan involve bystanders appropriately?
   - Did the plan demonstrate proper care?

Transparency Master 26

7. At the end of the lesson, answer any questions the participants still have. Make sure that each participant has an opportunity to resolve confusions or have questions answered.
8. Distribute a 20– to 25–question self-assessment exercise that you create from test bank questions. Explain to participants that they will review the exercise during the next lesson.

Assignment:

◆ Complete self-assessment exercise 1.

Putting It All Together: Scenarios

Scenario 1
Conscious Person, Difficulty Breathing

Transparency Master 22

At work, you are summoned to assist a fellow worker who has been injured in a five-foot fall from a ladder. As you arrive, you notice the person sitting on the ground, writhing in pain and having trouble breathing as he clutches his arm to his chest. You want to help. How do you proceed?

Note: Because the victim is conscious, the participant should begin by talking to him. When the victim responds, the participant should realize that the victim has an open airway, is breathing, and has a pulse. The participant should scan the body to check for any severe bleeding. At this point, the primary survey is complete. The participant should continue by doing a secondary survey, beginning by questioning the injured person to determine how he fell and where he was hurt. The participant should proceed to check vital signs and finish with the head-to-toe examination. The participant should be careful not to aggravate any injury. The participant should speak in a calm, reassuring manner. Once breathing difficulty is evident, EMS personnel should be summoned.

Scenario 2
Unconscious Person, Breathing

Transparency Master 22

A frantic neighbor is knocking at your door. She says that she cannot wake her sleeping roommate. She remembers that her roommate took some pills about two hours ago, but she is not sure what they were or where her roommate keeps them. You enter and see a woman lying face up on the couch but not moving. How do you proceed?

Note: The participant should begin with a check for consciousness. Next, he or she should open the airway and check for breathing. The participant should realize that the victim is breathing; therefore, she has a pulse. A quick scan does not reveal any bleeding. At this point, EMS personnel should be summoned. The participant should maintain an open airway and continue to monitor breathing. Because unconsciousness is considered a life-threatening emergency, a secondary survey is not needed.

Scenario 3
Unconscious Person, Not Breathing, Has a Pulse

Transparency Master 23

It's early morning, and you are taking a swim. The pool is almost deserted. Only two other people are swimming. When you finish, you realize you have to hurry or be late for class. As you enter the locker room, you are startled to see a body lying motionless on the damp floor next to a row of lockers. You recognize the older person as one who had been swimming laps in the lane next to you. You want to help. How do you proceed?

Note: The participant should begin with a check for consciousness. Next, he or she should shout for help to attract someone such as the lifeguard or any other swimmers. The participant should position the person appropriately. Next, he or she should open the airway and check for breathing. Finding the person not breathing, the participant should indicate that he or she would give two breaths, check the pulse, and check for severe bleeding. Finding a pulse and no bleeding, the participant should state that rescue breathing should be done, and the pulse monitored periodically until EMS personnel arrive. At some point in the scenario, have a bystander arrive. The participant should instruct the bystander to call EMS personnel. Because respiratory arrest is a life-threatening emergency, a secondary survey is not needed.

Scenario 4
Unconscious Person, Not Breathing, No Pulse

Transparency Master 24

Awakened in the early morning by your mother's scream, you rush to your parents' bedroom. There you find your father lying motionless on the floor. Your mother tells you that he had been feeling ill for several hours and had vomited. She says that he emerged from the bathroom clutching his chest and in apparent pain. He suddenly collapsed to the floor. You want to help. How do you proceed?

Note: The participant should begin by checking for consciousness. Next, he or she should position the person appropriately, open the airway, and check for breathing. Finding none, the participant should indicate that he or she would give two breaths and then check the pulse. Finding none, the participant should quickly scan the body for severe bleeding and indicate that CPR should be started. The participant should instruct his or her mother to call EMS personnel at this point, if the call has not been made already. Because cardiac arrest is a life-threatening emergency, a secondary survey is not needed.

Scenario 5
Unconscious Person, Breathing, With Severe Bleeding

Transparency Master 25

You witness a bicyclist struck by a car. The bicyclist is thrown from the bike, striking her head. The driver of the vehicle gets out to help. As you approach, you see the bicyclist lying on her side, twitching. Blood is spurting from the victim's thigh onto the pavement. You want to help. How do you proceed?

Note: The participant should begin by making the scene safe, then checking for consciousness. Since this scenario suggests the possibility of head or spine injury, the participant might check for breathing without moving the victim. If uncertain as to whether breathing is present, the participant should position the person appropriately, open the airway, and check breathing. With the knowledge that the person is breathing, the participant knows there is a pulse and should scan the body for severe bleeding. Heavy bleeding from the thigh should be controlled either by the participant or by a bystander who has been instructed by the participant to do so. EMS personnel should be summoned. The participant should continue to monitor the airway and breathing. Because severe bleeding is a life-threatening emergency, the secondary survey is not needed.

Lesson 16: PUTTING IT ALL TOGETHER II

Class assignment prior to this lesson: Complete self-assessment exercise 1.

Length: 45 minutes

Needed: Transparency masters 22 through 26; self-assessment 1 answer key; blankets or mats; manikins (optional); decontamination supplies

Goal Statement: Given a series of scenarios involving both life-threatening and non-life-threatening emergencies, participants should be able to make appropriate decisions for care and demonstrate proper first aid techniques.

YOU ARE THE CITIZEN RESPONDER (Con't.)

Time: 30 minutes

Activity:

1. Ask the groups that did not have an opportunity to present their scenario in the previous class to do so now.
2. Remind the participants that they should use the Emergency Action Principles to guide their responses.
3. Each scenario should take about 10 minutes to present and there should be class discussion.
4. After a group has role-played a specific scenario, initiate a discussion by asking the class to evaluate the group's response using the questions below.
5. **The Plan of Action**
   - Did the group's plan follow the Emergency Action Principles?
     - Survey the scene
     - Primary survey
     - Call EMS
     - Secondary survey
   - Did the plan involve bystanders appropriately?
   - Did the plan demonstrate proper care?
6. At the end of this activity, answer any questions that the participants may have. Make sure that each participant has an opportunity to resolve confusions or have questions answered.

Instructor Notes

Transparency Masters 22 through 26

Blankets or Mats

Manikins (optional)

Decontamination Supplies

REVIEW SELF-ASSESSMENT EXERCISE

Time: 15 minutes

Activity:

1. Ask the participants to get out their completed self-assessment exercises.
2. Ask each participant to read aloud one question and its answer. Have the participant include briefly his or her reason for thinking that this answer is correct. Explain that participants can ask the class for help if they do not know the answer to a particular question.
3. Proceed sequentially through each of the questions until all of the questions have been answered.

Self-assessment Answer Key

Assignment:

- Read Introduction to Injuries (Part IV).

Lesson 17: INJURIES

Class assignment prior to this lesson:	Read Introduction to Injuries (Part IV).
Length:	45 minutes
Needed:	Video; color transparency 1; transparency masters 27 through 29; Healthy Lifestyles Awareness Inventory
Goal Statement:	Participants will become familiar with how injuries occur, factors affecting injuries, and how best to prevent injuries.

LIFE-THREATENING EMERGENCIES REVIEW

Instructor Notes

Time: 5 minutes

Primary Points:

- Life-threatening emergencies are found and cared for during the primary survey.
- Life-threatening emergencies include a victim who—
  - Is unconscious.
  - Is not breathing.
  - Has no pulse.
  - Is bleeding severely.
- It is important to recognize and care for life-threatening emergencies as soon as possible. EMS personnel should be summoned immediately.
- Shock is the inevitable result of any significant illness or injury. Shock can become a life-threatening condition.
- Take steps to minimize shock in any emergency situation, regardless of whether or not the signals of shock are present.
- Conditions that are not an immediate threat to life are found and cared for during the secondary survey.
- A secondary survey is performed only if there are no life-threatening conditions.

Color Transparency 1

INJURY FACTS

Time: 25 minutes

Overview

Primary Points:

- Injuries are a significant health problem in the United States.
- Injuries like diseases, such as cancer, heart disease, or stroke, are a major contributor to deaths in the United States.

Transparency Master 27

- Injury is the leading cause of death and disability for people age 1 to 44 years.
- Motor vehicle collisions are the most common cause of injury-related deaths, followed by falls, poisonings, drownings, and fire-related incidents.

  Note: If possible, have some local statistics for your community. Local EMS/fire personnel can often give you information on items such as the number of motor vehicle collisions, injuries, fatalities, drownings, and fire-related incidents.

- Although the body is designed to resist injuries, statistics indicate that most people will have a significant injury at some time in their lives.
- Initiate a discussion by asking how many participants have experienced an injury.
- Ask the participants to describe what type of injury they had. Expect answers such as cuts, bruises, broken bones, burns.
- Ask the participants to provide examples of some common causes of injuries.

Video:

Show the video segment: *Injuries* (05:30). Stop the video at the pause point.

Note: If you choose not to show this video segment, provide a brief scenario that illustrates how injuries can occur.

How Injuries Occur

Primary Points:

- Five forms of energy cause damage to the body: mechanical, heat, electrical, chemical, and radiation.
- Mechanical energy causes the majority of all injuries. The others combined only account for about 25 percent.
- There are two basic types of injury—soft tissue injury and musculoskeletal injury.
- Ask the participants to give an example of an injury for each of the forces below:
  - A direct force that causes injury at the site of the impact (can cause bruises, cuts, fractures)
  - An indirect force that causes injury away from the site of impact (can cause damage to muscles, bones, joints, or internal organs)
  - Twisting forces (can cause fractures and joint injuries).
  - Contracting forces (can cause muscle injuries)

Factors Affecting Injuries

Primary Points:

Transparency Master 28

- Age, gender, environment, and the use or abuse of alcohol all affect the injury rate.
- Injuries are highest among people under the age of 45.
- Older adults and people age 15 to 24 have the highest rate of deaths from injury.
- Males are at greater risk than females for any type of injury. Males suffer fatal injuries 2.5 times more than females.
- Where you live, how your house is constructed, the type of heat used in your home, and the climate affect the degree of injury risk. For example, death rates from injury are twice as high in low-income areas as in high-income areas.
- Alcohol is a contributing factor in almost half of all fatally injured drivers. Over 40 percent of the deaths among the 15- to

19-year-old age group are the result of motor vehicle crashes. About half of these involve alcohol.

◆ A significant number of victims who die as a result of falls, drownings, fires, assaults, and suicides have a blood-alcohol content over the legal limit.

INJURY PREVENTION

Time: 15 minutes

Overview

Primary Points:

◆ Injuries, like disease, do not occur at random. Many are predictable, preventable events that result when people interact with the environment.

◆ Three general strategies for preventing injury include—
- Persuading people at risk to alter behavior.
- Requiring change by law.
- Providing automatic protection by product and environmental design.

Transparency Master 29

◆ Because high-risk groups are the most difficult to influence, the most successful injury prevention strategy is the built-in protection of product design.

Reducing Your Personal Injury Risk

◆ Three steps could significantly reduce your risk of personal injury:
- Know your risks. The Healthy Lifestyles Awareness Inventory should help you identify them.
- Change behaviors so you can decrease your risk of injuries.
- Think safety. Be alert for and avoid potentially harmful conditions or activities that increase your risk of injury.

Healthy Lifestyles Awareness Inventory

Healthy Lifestyles Awareness Inventory

- Ask the participants to review both the "Occupation and Recreation Safety" and "Home and Work Safety" sections of their completed Healthy Lifestyles Awareness Inventory.
- Share the class average for those sections of the inventory.
- Ask how many participants have targeted injury prevention as part of their behavior modification goals.
- Ask those who have targeted this item for their behavior modification how their efforts are progressing. Ask what they have found most difficult to change and what has been the easiest.
- Allow sufficient time for participant responses.

Assignment:

- Read Chapter 8.

Lesson 18: SOFT TISSUE INJURIES I

Class assignment prior to this lesson: Read Chapter 8.

Length: 45 minutes

Needed: Video; color transparencies 21 through 24; transparency master 30; Participant Progress Log; skill sheets; blankets or mats; gauze pads; roller bandages

Goal Statement: The participants will become familiar with how to care for soft tissue injuries and demonstrate how to control bleeding.

SOFT TISSUE INJURIES

Instructor Notes

Time: 10 minutes

Review Soft Tissue Structures

Primary Points:

- Soft tissues include the layers of skin, fat, and muscle.
- The skin has two primary layers: superficial (epidermis) and deep (dermis).
- The superficial layer provides a barrier to bacteria and other organisms that can cause infections.
- The deep layer contains the important structures of the nerves, the sweat and oil glands, and the blood vessels.

Color Transparency 21

Wounds

Primary Points:

- Wounds are classified as either open or closed.
- A wound is closed when the soft tissue damage occurs beneath the surface of the skin, leaving the outer layer intact.
- A wound is open if there is a break in the skin's outer layer.
- Open wounds result in various amounts of bleeding.
- There are four common types of open wounds: abrasions, lacerations, avulsions, and punctures.
- An abrasion is characterized by skin that has been rubbed or scraped away.

Color Transparencies 21 through 24

- A laceration is a cut, usually from a sharp object. It can have either jagged or smooth edges.
- An avulsion is an injury in which a portion of the skin and sometimes other soft tissue is partially or completely torn away.
- A puncture wound results when the skin is pierced with a pointed object, such as a nail, a piece of glass, a splinter, or a knife.

Caring for Closed Wounds

Primary Points:

Transparency Master 30

- Most closed wounds do not require medical care.
- Direct pressure, elevation, and cold decrease bleeding in the area and help control swelling and pain.
- When applying ice or a chemical cold pack, place a gauze pad, towel, or other cloth between the ice and the skin.
- Be aware of possible serious injuries to internal structures such as bones, muscles, or organs.
- If a person complains of severe pain or cannot move a body part without pain, or if you think the force that caused the injury was great enough to cause a serious injury, seek medical attention immediately.

Caring for Major Open Wounds

Primary Points:

- A major open wound is one with severe bleeding, with a deep destruction of tissue, or with a deeply embedded impaled object.
- Do not waste time washing the wound.
- Apply clean dressings such as gauze pads.
- Control bleeding using direct pressure and elevation.
- Apply a bandage over the dressings to maintain pressure on the wound.
- Wash your hands immediately after giving care.
- Have the victim seek medical attention.

- If the victim has an impaled object in the wound—
  - Do not remove the object.
  - Use bulky dressings to stabilize it.
  - Control bleeding by bandaging the dressing in place around the object.

Caring for Minor Open Wounds

Primary Points:

- A minor wound is one in which damage is only superficial and bleeding is minimal.
- Wash the wound thoroughly with soap and water.
- Place a sterile dressing over the wound.
- Apply direct pressure for a few minutes to control bleeding.
- Once bleeding is controlled, remove the dressing and apply an antibiotic ointment.
- Apply a new dressing, such as an adhesive bandage.

BLEEDING CONTROL

Time: 15 minutes

Video:

Show the video: *Controlling Bleeding* (09:00). Stop the video at the pause point. Address any questions participants may have.

Note: If you choose not to show the video, demonstrate how to control bleeding. Make sure all participants can see the demonstration.

Primary Points:

- A dressing is a pad placed directly over a wound to absorb blood and other body fluids and to prevent infection.
- A bandage is any material used to wrap or cover a part of the body. It is commonly used to hold dressings in place, to apply pressure to control bleeding, to protect a wound from dirt and infection, and to provide support to an injured limb or body part.

- Two commonly used bandages are the adhesive and roller bandage types. Other common bandages, such as a triangular bandage and a cravat bandage, will be discussed in more detail in Chapter 9.
- To apply a roller bandage—
  - Elevate the injured part, if possible.
  - Secure the end of the bandage.
  - Completely cover the dressings using overlapping turns.
- Do not cover fingers or toes, if possible.
- If blood soaks through, apply additional dressings and another bandage.

SKILL PRACTICE: CONTROLLING BLEEDING

Time: 20 minutes

Activity:

1. Move the participants into the practice area.
2. Ask the participants to get a partner.
3. Explain to the participants that they will practice controlling bleeding on each other.
4. Guide the participants through the skill. Watch participants as they practice, giving help when appropriate or when requested.
5. After participants have practiced the skills to the point at which they feel comfortable in their ability to perform them, have the participants change places. Repeat the practice. Check participants' skills as you watch them practice.
6. Answer any questions that participants may have.

Skill Sheets

Gauze Pads

Roller Gauze

Blanket or Mats

Participant Progress Log

Assignment:

- Read Chapter 9.

Lesson 19: SOFT TISSUE INJURIES II/ MUSCULOSKELETAL INJURIES I

Class assignment prior to this lesson: Read Chapter 9.

Length: 45 minutes

Needed: Video; color transparencies 10 through 13 and 25 through 36; transparency masters 31 through 33

Goal Statement: Participants will become familiar with how to provide care for burn injuries and how to recognize serious musculoskeletal injuries.

BURNS

Time: 15 minutes

Instructor Notes

Color Transparencies 25 and 26

Primary Points:

- Burns are another type of soft tissue injury, caused by heat, certain chemicals, electricity, solar radiation, or other forms of radiation.
- Burns are classified as superficial (outer layer), partial-thickness (both layers), or full-thickness (both layers of skin plus underlying structures such as fat and muscles).
- Severity of the burn depends on—
  - Temperature of the object.
  - Length of exposure.
  - Location of the burn.
  - Extent of the burn.
  - Victim's age and medical condition.
- Superficial burns appear red and dry and are usually painful. The area may swell. They generally heal in a few days without scarring.
- Partial-thickness burns appear red and wet and have blisters that may open and weep clear fluid. These burns are usually painful, and the area often swells. They generally heal in three to four weeks, and scarring may occur.
- Full-thickness burns appear brown or charred (black), with the tissues underneath sometimes appearing white. They

can either be extremely painful or relatively painless if the burn destroyed nerve endings in the skin. Full-thickness burns take longer to heal and usually result in scarring.

- ◆ A critical burn is one that requires the attention of medical professionals. Critical burns are potentially life-threatening, disfiguring, or disabling.
- ◆ It is not always possible to determine the extent of damage caused by a burn immediately after the injury occurs.
- ◆ Some factors that can help you determine if a burn is critical include—
  - Burns whose victims are experiencing breathing difficulty.
  - Burns covering more than one body part.
  - Burns to the head, neck, hands, feet, or genitals.
  - Any partial-thickness or full-thickness burn to a child or an elderly person.
  - Burns resulting from chemicals, explosions, or electricity.
- ◆ Always call EMS personnel immediately for any burn you suspect is critical.

Care for Burns

Primary Points:

- ◆ Ensure that the scene is safe.
- ◆ Do a primary survey. Pay close attention to the victim's airway. Look for signs of burn injury around the face. If you suspect a burned airway or burned lungs, continually monitor breathing. Summon EMS personnel immediately.
- ◆ Look for additional signs of burns. If burns are present, follow these basic care steps:
  - Cool the burned area to stop the burning.
  - Cover the burned area to prevent infection.
  - Take steps to minimize shock.
- ◆ If the burn is caused by a chemical—whether on the skin or in the eyes—flush

Transparency Master 31

the burned area with large amounts of cool, running water for at least 10 minutes after the victim stops feeling pain or until EMS personnel arrive and take over. Have the victim remove contaminated clothes.

- Electrical burns can cause both serious internal and external injuries.
- To care for a victim of an electrical burn—
  - Make sure the scene is safe. Turn off any electrical current before approaching victim.
  - Do a primary survey and care for life-threatening emergencies such as unconsciousness, or respiratory or cardiac arrest.
  - In the secondary survey, look for two burn sites. These are entry and exit wounds indicating where electricity passed through the body.
  - Take steps to minimize shock.

MUSCULOSKELETAL INJURIES

Time: 10 minutes

Overview

Primary Points:

- Musculoskeletal injuries are often painful but are rarely life-threatening.
- When not recognized and taken care of properly, they can have serious consequences and even result in permanent disability.
- Developing a better understanding of the structure and functions of the body's framework will help you better assess musculoskeletal injuries and give appropriate care.

Review of Anatomy

Primary Points:

- The body has over 600 muscles. Most are skeletal muscles, which attach to the bones.

Color Transparencies 10 through 13, and 27 through 32

- Unlike other soft tissues, muscles are able to contract and relax. These actions are responsible for all body movements.
- Through a pathway of nerves, the brain directs muscles to move.
- Motion is usually caused by a group of muscles close together, pulling at the same time.
- Injuries to the brain, the spinal cord, or the nerves can affect muscle control. A loss of muscle control is called paralysis.
- The skeleton is formed by over 200 bones of various sizes and shapes.
- The skeleton protects vital organs and other soft tissues.
- Two or more bones come together to form joints. Ligaments hold bones together at joints.
- Bones are hard, dense tissues with a rich supply of blood and nerves.
- The bony structures that form the skeleton define the parts of the body. The head is formed by the bones that form the skull, the chest is defined by the bones that form the rib cage, and so on.

Injuries to the Musculoskeletal System

Primary Points:

- There are four basic types of musculoskeletal injuries—fracture, dislocation, sprain, and strain.
- Injuries can be classified according to the body structures that are damaged.
  - A fracture is a break or disruption in bone.
  - Fractures are classified as open or closed.
  - A dislocation is a displacement or separation of a bone from its normal position at a joint.
  - A sprain is the partial or complete tearing of ligaments and other tissues at a joint.
  - A strain is a stretching and tearing of muscle or tendon fibers.

Color Transparencies 33 through 35

RECOGNIZING MUSCULOSKELETAL INJURIES

Time: 5 minutes

Common Signals

Primary Points:

- Identify and care for injuries to the musculoskeletal system during the secondary survey.
- It is not easy to determine exactly what type of injury a victim has.
- Five common signals of musculoskeletal injury include—
  - Pain.
  - Swelling.
  - Deformity
  - Discoloration of the skin.
  - Limited use of the injured body part.

Transparency Master 32

Signals of Serious Injury

Primary Points:

- Five common signals of **serious** musculo-skeletal injury include—
  - Significant deformity.
  - Inability to move or use the affected body part.
  - Bone fragments protruding from wound.
  - Bones grating or a snap or pop felt or heard by the victim.
  - A cause of injury that suggests the injury may be severe.
- Call EMS personnel immediately if—
  - The injury impairs breathing.
  - You see or suspect multiple musculoskeletal injuries.

CARING FOR MUSCULOSKELETAL INJURIES

Time: 15 minutes

Video:

Show the video segment: *Splinting* (09:30). Stop the video at the pause point. Address any questions participants may have.

Note: If you choose not to show the video, demonstrate splinting a forearm, a leg, and an ankle. Make sure that all participants can see the demonstration.

General Care

Primary Points:

- Rest the injured body part. Avoid any movements or activities that cause pain. Help the victim find the most comfortable position. If you suspect head or spine injuries, leave the victim lying flat.
- Apply ice or a cold pack to the injured area. Cold packs help reduce swelling and ease pain and discomfort. Place a layer of gauze or cloth between the source of cold and the skin to prevent damage to the skin.
- Elevate the injured part if doing so does not cause further injury. Do not attempt to elevate a fractured part until it has been splinted.
- Immobilize any musculoskeletal injury you suspect is serious.

Transparency Master 33

Color Transparency 36

Assignment:

- Review Chapter 9 skill sheets: Splinting (pages 222 through 227).
- Read Chapters 10 through 12.

Lesson 20: MUSCULOSKELETAL INJURIES II

Class assignment prior to this lesson:	Review Chapter 9 skill sheets: Splinting (pages 222 through 227). Read Chapters 10 through 12.
Length:	45 minutes
Needed:	Participant Progress Log; skill sheets; blankets; triangular bandages; rigid splints
Goal Statement:	Participants should become familiar with different methods of immobilizing injured body parts.

SKILL PRACTICE: SPLINTING

Time: 45 minutes

Activity:

1. Move the participants into the practice area.
2. Assign partners or ask the participants to find partners.
3. Ask participants to apply a rigid splint to the forearm and then apply a sling and binder.
4. Watch the participants as they practice, giving help when appropriate or requested.
5. After participants have practiced the skills to the point at which they feel comfortable in their ability to perform them, have the participants change places. Repeat the practice. Check participants' skills as you watch them practice.
6. Ask participants to apply an anatomic splint to the leg. Repeat the practice and skill check.
7. Ask participants to apply a soft splint to the ankle. Repeat the practice and skill check.
8. Answer any questions that participants may have.
9. Briefly review the several steps of care for any musculoskeletal injury.

Instructor Notes

Skill Sheets,

Participant Progress Log

Blankets

Triangular Bandages

Splinting Devices

Assignment:

- Review Chapters 10 through 12.

Lesson 21: SPECIFIC INJURIES

Class assignment prior to this lesson: Review Chapters 10 through 12.

Length: 45 minutes

Needed: Color transparencies 36 through 42; transparency masters 34 through 38

Goal Statement: Participants should become familiar with how specific injuries to the head, spine, chest, abdomen, and (sometimes) extremities can result in serious musculoskeletal injuries.

INJURIES TO THE HEAD AND SPINE

Time: 25 minutes

Instructor Notes

Overview

Primary Points:

- Although injuries to the head and spine account for a small percentage of all injuries, they cause more than half of the fatalities. **Color Transparency 37**
- Motor vehicle collisions account for about half of all head and spine injuries. Other causes include falls, sports and recreational activities, and violent acts such as assaults.
- Nearly 80,000 victims are permanently disabled each year in America as a result of head and spine injuries.
- Prompt care can prevent some head and spine injuries from becoming more serious.
- Injuries to the head and spine can damage both bone (skull, vertebrae) and soft tissue (brain, spinal cord). **Color Transparency 38**

Common Causes of Serious Head/Spine Injury

Primary Points:

- Consider the possibility of a serious head or spine injury in—
  - A fall from a height greater than the victim's height.
  - Any motor vehicle collision.

- A person found unconscious for unknown reasons.
- Any injury involving severe blunt force to the head or trunk.
- Any injury that penetrates the head or trunk.
- A motor vehicle crash involving a driver or passengers not wearing safety belts.
- Any person thrown from a motor vehicle.
- Any injury in which a victim's helmet is broken, including a motorcycle, football, or industrial helmet.

Signals of Serious Head and Spine Injury

Primary Points:

Transparency Master 34

- ◆ Signals of a serious head or spine injury may be slow to develop.
- ◆ Signals of a serious head or spine injury include—
  - Changes in level of consciousness.
  - Severe pain or pressure in the head, neck, or back.
  - Tingling or loss of sensation in the extremities.
  - Partial or complete loss of movement of any body parts.
  - Unusual bumps or depressions on the head or spine.
  - Blood or other fluids in the ears or nose.
  - Profuse external bleeding of the head, neck, or back.
  - Seizures.
  - Impaired breathing or vision as a result of injury.
  - Nausea or vomiting.
  - Persistent headache.
  - Loss of balance.
  - Bruising of the head, especially around the eyes or the back of the head.

Caring for Head and Spine Injuries

Primary Points:

- Head and spine injuries can become life-threatening or severely disabling emergencies.
- While waiting for EMS personnel to arrive, always care for head and spine injuries as follows:
  - Minimize movement of the head and spine.
  - Maintain an open airway.
  - Monitor consciousness and breathing.
  - Control any external bleeding.
  - Maintain normal body temperature.
- Excessive movement of the head and spine can damage the spinal cord irreversibly. Keep the victim as still as possible, using the technique called in-line stabilization.
- Explain that in-line stabilization is done by simply placing your hands on both sides of the victim's head. Gently position the head, if necessary, in line with the body, and support it in that position until EMS personnel arrive.
- Explain that this can be done for victims in many positions: lying down, sitting, or standing.
- Certain circumstances require that you do not move the victim's head in line with the body:
  - When the victim's head is severely angled.
  - When the victim complains of pain, pressure, or muscle spasms on initial movement of the head.
  - When the rescuer feels resistance when attempting to move the head.

  In these circumstances, support the victim's head in the position in which it is found.
- Checking for breathing does not always require rolling the victim onto his or her back. A cry of pain, chest movement, or the sound of breathing tells you the

victim is breathing. If the victim vomits, carefully roll the victim onto one side to keep the airway clear. This is more easily done by two people.

- A victim of serious head or spine injury will experience changes in consciousness. The victim may give inappropriate responses to name, time, place, or what happened. He or she may speak incoherently. The victim may appear drowsy, appear suddenly to lapse into sleep and then awaken, or lose consciousness completely. Breathing may become rapid or irregular. Breathing may also stop if chest nerves or the spinal cord are damaged.
- Control bleeding with direct pressure and pressure bandages.
- Because a serious head or spine injury can result in a disruption of the body's heating and cooling mechanism, a victim of such injury is more susceptible to shock. Maintain normal body temperature.

Activity:

1. Ask participants and their partners to practice the proper positioning of a victim by using the in-line stabilization technique.
2. Have participants act as seated victims involved in a vehicle collision. Have rescuers stabilize the victim's head or neck, either from behind, beside, or in front of the victim.
3. When participants have practiced and feel competent in performing the skill, have them change positions with their partners. Repeat the practice. (There is no skill check for in-line stabilization.)
4. Answer any questions participants may have.

INJURIES TO THE CHEST, ABDOMEN, AND PELVIS

Time: 15 minutes

CHEST INJURY

Signals of Serious Chest Injury

Primary Points:

- Signals of serious chest injury include—
  - Difficulty breathing.
  - Severe pain.
  - Discoloration.
  - Deformity.
  - Coughing up blood.
- If the victim is coughing up blood, it could indicate a serious injury to the lung(s).
- Sometimes this injury to the lung(s) is caused by an object penetrating the chest cavity.
- Penetrating injuries can sometimes result in "sucking chest wounds." These are wounds that make a distinctive "sucking" sound as the person breathes.

Transparency Master 35

Color Transparency 39

Color Transparency 40

Caring for Serious Chest Injury

Primary Points:

- Caring for serious chest injury often means helping the victim to overcome breathing difficulty.
- Position the victim to aid breathing.
- If ribs are broken, binding the victim's arm to the injured side can help support the injured area and make breathing easier.
- If a sucking chest sound is evident, cover the wound with an airtight dressing such as plastic wrap. Tape it in place, leaving only one corner uncovered.
- Call EMS personnel.

ABDOMINAL INJURY

Signals of Serious Abdominal Injury

Primary Points:

- Like chest injuries, signals of serious abdominal injuries include pain and discoloration. Other signals are—
  - Nausea and vomiting.
  - Thirst.

Transparency Master 36

Color Transparency 39

- Rigid abdomen.
- Weakness.
- Organs protruding from the abdomen.

Caring for Serious Abdominal Injury

Primary Points:

- ◆ If the injury involves an open wound—
  - **Do not** put pressure on any protruding organs or try to put them back inside.
  - Position the victim on his or her back.
  - Cover the wound loosely with moist, clean dressings.
  - Place plastic wrap over the dressings and lightly cover with a towel to help maintain warmth.
- ◆ If the injury involves a closed wound—
  - Position the victim on his or her back.
  - Try bending the victim's knees slightly, placing pillows or blankets under the legs for support.
- ◆ Whether they are open or closed, abdominal injuries should be cared for by medical professionals, since shock is likely to occur with a serious injury.
- ◆ Even if shock were occurring, you have already taken steps to minimize it by properly positioning the victim.

PELVIC INJURY

Signals of Serious Pelvic Injury

Primary Points:

- ◆ Signals are the same as those of abdominal injury, with the addition of—
  - Loss of sensation or movement in the legs (sometimes occurs).

Color Transparency 41

Transparency Master 37

Caring for Pelvic Injury

Primary Points:

- ◆ Care for pelvic injuries by minimizing movement of the victim.
- ◆ Since pelvic injuries sometimes involve the genitals, pain can be severe.
- ◆ If an open wound to the genital area is present, control any bleeding with direct pressure.
- ◆ Summon EMS personnel immediately for any pelvic injury.

INJURIES TO THE EXTREMITIES

Time: 5 minutes

Overview

Primary Points:

- Injuries can range from a simple bruise on the arm to a life-threatening injury involving severe bleeding, such as the bleeding that may occur with a fractured femur.

Signals of Serious Extremity Injury

Primary Points:

- Signals include—
  - Pain.
  - Tenderness.
  - Swelling.
  - Discoloration (such as bruising).
  - Deformity.
  - Inability to use the limb.
  - Loss of sensation.
  - A limb that is cold to the touch.
  - Severe external bleeding.

Color Transparency 42

Transparency Master 38

Caring for Serious Extremity Injury

Primary Points:

- Care involves immobilizing the injured area as best you can. Splint the area so that movement is restricted above and below the injury site.
- Ice applied to the injured area can help reduce pain and swelling.
- EMS personnel should be contacted for any injury involving weight-bearing bones (thigh, leg, ankle) because someone with this type of injury will have difficulty being transported to a hospital since they are often unable to walk.

Color Transparency 36

Lesson Summary

- Summarize the lesson by reinforcing that care for any injury involves the following:
  - Do a primary survey, and care for any life-threatening conditions caused by the injury. Always start with the ABCs.
  - Be gentle as you provide care for specific injuries.

- Minimize movement.
- Call EMS personnel for help.

Assignment:

- Review Chapters 8 through 12 and complete unanswered Study Questions.

Lesson 22: PUTTING IT ALL TOGETHER I

Class assignment prior to this lesson:	Review Chapters 8 through 12 and complete unanswered Study Questions.
Length:	45 minutes
Needed:	Color transparency 1; transparency masters 26 and 39 through 41; blankets or mats; manikins (optional); decontamination supplies; various splinting devices; triangular bandages, roller gauze, gauze pads; self-assessment exercise 2
Goal Statement:	Given a series of scenarios involving injury that results in either life-threatening or non-life-threatening conditions, participants should be able to make appropriate decisions regarding care and demonstrate proper first aid techniques.

YOU ARE THE CITIZEN RESPONDER

Time: 45 minutes

Activity:

1. Divide the participants into small groups. Give each group one of the "Putting It All Together" scenarios (see pages 129 through 132 in this manual.)
2. Tell the participants they will be given 10 minutes to decide how best to respond to the emergency situation they have been given.

   Note: Tell participants that they are expected to be able to discuss/demonstrate any previously learned skill that is required to respond effectively. If the group feels it is necessary to use a skill they have not learned (such as movement of a victim from a dangerous area), they may simply explain their actions, and will not be required to demonstrate it.

3. Remind the participants that they should use the Emergency Action Principles to guide their responses.
4. After 10 minutes, ask each group to present their scenario to the rest of the class. Each scenario should take about 10 minutes.

Instructor Notes

Blankets or Mats

Manikins (optional)

Decontamination Supplies

Splinting Devices

Triangular Bandages

Roller Gauze

Gauze Pads

Color Transparency 1

5. One at a time, use the transparencies or have participants read the scenario aloud to the class and role-play their response to their emergency. Tell the participants that they should demonstrate any previously learned skill that would be required as an effective response.

   At any time during the role play, they may choose to use either a manikin or a member of the group as the victim. Each group should discuss their actions while giving care. They should also be able to answer questions the instructor or other participants may have.

Transparency Masters 39 through 41

6. After a group has role-played a specific scenario, initiate a discussion by asking the class to evaluate the group's response, using the questions below.

   Note: It is unlikely that all groups will be able to present scenarios during this class. Time has been allowed for remaining groups in the next lesson.

   The Plan of Action

   Transparency Master 26

   - Did the group's plan follow the Emergency Action Principles?
     - Survey the scene
     - Primary survey
     - Call EMS
     - Secondary survey
   - Did the plan involve bystanders appropriately?
   - Did the plan demonstrate proper care?
   - In addition, ask what specific signals the group noticed and what type of injury they might suspect.

7. At the end of the lesson, ask the participants what questions they have. Make sure that the participants have an opportunity to resolve their confusions or have their questions answered.
8. Distribute the 20– to 25–question self-assessment exercise 2 that you create from the test bank questions. Explain to

participants that they will review the exercise during the next lesson.

Assignment:

- Complete self-assessment exercise 2.

Putting It All Together: Scenarios

Scenario 1
Conscious Person, Serious Head and Spine Injury

Transparency Master 39

At work, you are summoned to assist another employee who has been injured in an eight-foot fall from a ladder. As you arrive, you see the person lying on the ground. She is crying and moaning in pain. A bystander says that she landed on her back. The victim has not moved from this position. She says that she has tingling and numbness in her legs and feet and pain in her back. She also has a two-inch laceration on the side of her head. You want to help. How do you proceed?

Note: Participants should first check to see that the scene is safe. Make sure nothing is going to fall—objects such as lights, boxes, or whatever the worker was dealing with while on the ladder. Since the victim is conscious, the participants should begin by talking to the victim. The victim's verbal responses assure that her airway is open, she is breathing, and has a pulse. Bleeding from the side of the head should be controlled with direct pressure and in-line stabilization maintained. The secondary survey could reveal any developing signals of shock. Since the "mechanism of injury" suggests a serious head and spine injury, notify EMS personnel immediately and take steps to minimize shock, such as monitoring ABCs, keeping the person lying flat, and maintaining normal body temperature until EMS personnel arrive.

Scenario 2
Multiple Victims, Serious Extremity Injuries

Transparency Master 40

You and a friend are driving home and see a collision between a bicyclist and skateboarder. Both are thrown to the pavement. Both are conscious and in pain. The skateboarder was struck on the outside of his leg by the bike. The leg is bent, and his knee has an obvious deformity. The bicyclist was thrown over the handle bars, landing on her outstretched arms. She is bleeding from abrasions on both forearms and her wrist has an obvious deformity. You have a first aid kit in your car. You want to help. How do you proceed?

Note: Participants should first make sure the scene is safe, then begin talking to the victims. The victims' verbal responses ensure that there is an open airway, breathing, and pulse. The secondary survey would provide a quick check for other injuries. By shouting for help, you might attract other bystanders who could call EMS personnel. Bleeding from the bicyclist's arms should be controlled, and both victims' injured extremities immobilized in the position the participants found them, using whatever supplies participants have available.

Scenario 3
Conscious Victim, Extremity Injury

You are coaching a Little League baseball team. The pitcher is struck with a line drive to the ankle and falls to the ground. He is crying and in pain, unable to move the limb. Slight swelling and discoloration are already present. You are about three minutes away from the nearest hospital. The player's parents are not at the game. You want to help. How do you proceed?

Note: Knowing that the scene is safe, the participant can proceed to help the injured player. Since he is crying, the airway is open, he is breathing, and has a pulse. The injured area should be immobilized, and ice or a cold pack applied to control the swelling, if possible. Whether to call EMS personnel for assistance or to transport the child yourself is a difficult decision. It will be based on several factors: Is an additional coach available—to transport the injured pitcher, or to continue coaching the other members of the team while you transport the player? Is a phone available to call EMS personnel? Is it possible to move the player into a vehicle without aggravating the injury further? Can the parents be reached?

Scenario 4

Conscious Victim, Multiple Injuries

Transparency Master 41

On a cool fall day, you and a group of friends are hiking through a state park. The terrain you have chosen is rough, with a few steep inclines. After you have been hiking about an hour, suddenly one of the hikers loses his footing and tumbles approximately 30 feet down a steep slope. He strikes several rocks along the way. You and another hiker are able to make your way down to the victim quickly and safely. The victim appears to have been temporarily unconscious. While he is now conscious, he is dazed and unsure of his surroundings. There is a large bruise on his forehead. He says that he cannot move one of his arms. His elbow is bruised, swollen, and bleeding. He also has a stick approximately four inches long and one inch wide impaled in his hand. You have first aid supplies in your backpack. You want to help. How do you proceed?

Note: With the scene safe, one of the participants should stabilize the head and spine. This same person should talk with the victim, monitoring consciousness and ABCs. The second participant should apply a cold compress (if instant cold pack is available) to the forehead, control bleeding at the elbow, immobilize the elbow, and bandage the hand in a manner that restricts movement of the impaled object. Two other bikers in the group should be sent to the nearest ranger station, telephone, or road to get assistance. Further care for the victim should include minimizing total body movement and maintaining normal body temperature by using whatever clothing is available until rescue personnel can arrive. Any remaining bikers can help mark the location of the victim and rescuers on the trail (using such objects as clothing, backpacks, or flagging tape) to make it easier for arriving rescue personnel to locate them.

Lesson 23: PUTTING IT ALL TOGETHER II

Class assignment prior to this lesson: Complete self-assessment exercise 2.

Length: 45 minutes

Needed: Transparency masters 26, 39 through 41; self-assessment 2 answer key; blankets or mats; manikins (optional); decontamination supplies; various splinting devices; triangular bandages, roller gauze and gauze pads

Goal Statement: Given a series of scenarios involving both life-threatening and non-life-threatening conditions, participants should be able to make appropriate decisions regarding care and demonstrate proper first aid techniques.

YOU ARE THE CITIZEN RESPONDER (Con't.) Instructor Notes

Time: 30 minutes

Activity:

1. Tell the groups that did not have an opportunity to present their scenario earlier that they will do so now.
2. Remind the participants that they should use the Emergency Action Principles to guide their responses.
3. Each scenario should take about ten minutes to present.
4. After a group has role-played a specific scenario, initiate a discussion by asking the class to evaluate the group's response, using the questions below.

The Plan of Action

- Did the plan of action follow the Emergency Action Principles?
  - Survey the scene
  - Primary survey
  - Call EMS
  - Secondary survey
- Did the plan involve bystanders appropriately?
- Did the plan demonstrate proper care?

5. At the end of this activity, answer any questions that the participants have.

Transparency Masters 39 through 41

Blankets or Mats

Manikins (optional)

Decontamination Supplies

Splinting Devices

Triangular Bandages

Roller Gauze

Gauze Pads

Transparency Master 26

Make sure that participants have an opportunity to resolve their confusions or have their questions answered.

REVIEW SELF-ASSESSMENT EXERCISE

Time: 15 minutes

Activity:

Self-Assessment Exercise 2

Self-assessment Answer Key

1. Ask the participants to get out their completed self-assessment exercises.
2. Ask each participant to read aloud one question and its answer. Have participants include a very brief reason for why they think the answer is correct. Explain that participants can ask the class for help if they do not know the answer to a particular question.
3. Proceed sequentially through each of the questions until all have been answered.

Assignment:

- Read the Introduction to Part V: Medical Emergencies.
- Read Chapters 13 and 14.

Lesson 24: MEDICAL EMERGENCIES

Class assignment prior to this lesson:	Read the Introduction to Part V: Medical Emergencies. Read Chapters 13 and 14.
Length:	45 minutes
Needed:	Video; color transparencies 43 through 47; transparency masters 42 through 49; flip chart or chalkboard
Goal Statement:	Participants will become familiar with the signals of medical emergencies and how to give appropriate care.

RESPONDING TO A MEDICAL EMERGENCY

Instructor Notes

Time: 15 minutes

Primary Points:

- Explain to participants that medical emergencies often cause both a great deal of confusion on the part of rescuers and lost time in summoning professionals. This need not be the case.

Video:

Show the video segment: *Medical Emergencies* (06:00). Stop the video at the next pause point. Address any questions participants may have.

Note: If you do not have the video, use the entire 15 minutes on the following activity.

Activity:

1. Ask the participants how many of them have experienced a situation in which someone has become suddenly ill.
2. Ask some of the participants to share with the class what happened, how they felt, and how the victims were cared for.
3. Record on a flip chart or chalkboard the signals the victim displayed or described.
4. Explain that certain illnesses occur suddenly. Others may develop over a period of time, such as a diabetic emergency. They all display some type of signals.

Flip Chart/ Chalkboard

5. Sudden illnesses often show the following signals:
   - Change in a person's level of consciousness
   - Complaint of feeling light-headed, dizzy, or weak
   - Complaint of feeling nauseated, or the victim may vomit
   - Breathing, pulse, or skin temperature, color, and/or moisture may change.
6. The fact that someone looks and feels ill indicates that there is a problem.
   - You do not need to know the cause of the sudden illness in order to provide appropriate care for the victim.

Color Transparency 43

SPECIFIC SUDDEN ILLNESS

Time: 15 minutes

Primary Points:

- ◆ Some common sudden illnesses include—
  - Fainting, diabetic emergencies, seizures, stroke, poisoning, and the previously discussed heart attack.
- ◆ Tell participants to notice how, as you go through these specific illnesses, they all exhibit some of the generic signals listed above.

Transparency Master 42

Fainting

Primary Points:

- ◆ Fainting is a common sudden illness characterized by partial or complete loss of consciousness.
- ◆ Fainting is caused by a temporary reduction of blood flow to the brain.
- ◆ Since fainting is actually one type of shock, the victim will commonly display shocklike signals such as dizziness; nausea; and cool, moist, pale skin.
- ◆ Fainting usually resolves by itself when normal blood flow to the brain is restored, for example when the person is in a horizontal position.

Transparency Master 43

- Fainting by itself does not usually harm the victim, but injury may occur from falling.
- Position the person on a flat surface. If possible, elevate the legs 8 to 12 inches. Check ABCs. Loosen any restrictive clothing. Do not give the victim anything to eat or drink, or splash water in the victim's face. Since you cannot be certain why a person has fainted, call EMS personnel.

Diabetic Emergency

Primary Points:

- Insulin is a hormone that takes the sugar from the bloodstream to the cells where it is used.
- The condition in which the body does not produce enough insulin is called diabetes mellitus. A person with this condition is a diabetic.
- Anyone with diabetes must carefully monitor his or her diet and exercise. Insulin-dependent diabetics must also regulate their use of insulin.
- When a diabetic fails to control these factors, one of two problems can occur—too much or too little sugar in the bloodstream. This imbalance causes illness.
- Hyperglycemia means too much sugar. Consequently, the insulin level is too low. Without insulin, body cells cannot get the sugar they need, even though there is abundant sugar present. To meet its energy needs, the body will break down other food sources. This results in a person becoming ill over a period of time, as excess waste products build up in the body. This condition can result in a serious form of diabetic emergency—diabetic coma.

Color Transparency 44

- On the other hand, too little sugar can be present. This is hypoglycemia. Consequently, the insulin level is too high. The small amount of sugar remaining is used

Transparency Master 44

rapidly. When the brain gets too little sugar to function, it results in an acute condition called insulin reaction.

- ◆ Whether too much or too little sugar, both can result in a diabetic emergency. The main signals of a diabetic emergency include—
  - Changes in levels of consciousness.
  - Rapid breathing and pulse.
  - Feeling and looking ill.
- ◆ It is not important to differentiate between the two conditions. To provide care—
  - Care for any life-threatening conditions you find.
  - If victim is conscious and there are no life-threatening conditions, do a secondary survey. Look for a medical alert tag, or ask if victim has a medical condition (such as diabetes). If the victim is a diabetic and he or she is exhibiting signals of a diabetic emergency, care for it as such.
  - If conscious and able to swallow, give the victim sugar in form of fruit juices, candy or nondiet soft drinks. If the victim's condition is caused by low sugar, the sugar you give will help quickly. If caused by high sugar, the excess sugar will do no further harm.
  - If the person is unconscious, do not give anything by mouth. Monitor the ABCs and maintain normal body temperature. Call EMS personnel because unconsciousness is a serious condition.

Seizures

Primary Points:

- ◆ When normal functions of the brain are disrupted by injury, disease, fever, or infection, the electrical activity of the brain becomes irregular. This irregularity can cause a sudden loss of body control known as seizure.

- The chronic form of seizure is known as epilepsy. Although epilepsy is usually controlled with medication, some people with epilepsy have seizures from time to time.
- Before a seizure occurs, the person may experience a warning called an aura. This is an unusual sensation or feeling such as a visual hallucination; a strange sound, taste, or smell; or an urgent need to get to safety.

Transparency Master 45

- Seizure may range from mild blackouts that others mistake for daydreaming to sudden uncontrolled muscular contractions lasting several minutes.
- Do not try to stop the seizure or restrain the person. Protect the person from injury and manage the airway. Remove nearby objects and protect the person's head. If there is fluid such as saliva, blood, or vomit in the person's mouth, position him or her on one side so that the fluid drains from the mouth.
- Do not place anything between the teeth.
- When the seizure is over, the person will be drowsy and disoriented. Do a secondary survey to check and care for any injuries. Be reassuring and comforting.
- EMS personnel should be called if—
    - The seizure lasts more than a few minutes.
    - The victim has repeated seizures.
    - The victim appears to be injured.
    - You are uncertain about the cause of the seizure.
    - The victim is pregnant.
    - The victim is a known diabetic.
    - The victim is an infant or child.
    - The seizure takes place in water.
    - The victim fails to regain consciousness.

Transparency Master 46

Stroke

Primary Points:

- A stroke is a disruption of blood flow to a part of the brain that is serious enough to cause brain damage.
- It is most commonly caused by a blood clot that forms or lodges in the arteries that supply blood to the brain. Another cause is bleeding from a ruptured artery in the brain.
- A transient ischemic attack (TIA) is a temporary episode that is like a stroke—sometimes called a "mini-stroke." Like a stroke, TIA results in reduced blood flow to the brain.
- A victim of stroke will appear or feel ill or will exhibit abnormal behavior. Signals include sudden weakness and numbness of the face, arm, or leg, often on only one side of the body. The victim may have difficulty talking or understanding speech. Vision may be blurred or dimmed; pupils may be unequal in size; the victim may experience a sudden severe headache, dizziness, confusion, ringing in the ears, or lose consciousness.
- Like other sudden illnesses, priority involves caring for ABCs. If there is fluid or vomit in the victim's mouth, position him or her on one side to allow any fluids to drain out of the mouth. You may have to clear the airway of debris with your finger. Call EMS personnel immediately, and monitor ABCs until they arrive.

Color Transparency 45

Transparency Master 47

POISONING

Time: 15 minutes

Poisoning Facts

Primary Points:

- Poisoning is also a sudden illness. What makes it unique is that this sudden illness is brought on by external substances entering the body.
- Upwards of 2 million poisonings occur each year in the United States.

Note: If desired, check with local hospitals or Poison Control Center to get statistics on the number and types of poisonings in your particular area.

- The majority of poisonings occur in the home.
- Poisoning fatalities among adults (especially older adults) have been increasing over the last decade due to increases in poisoning-related suicides and drug-related poisonings, including both illegal drugs and prescribed medications.

Methods of Poisoning

Activity:

1. Ask participants how poisons enter the body. Ask for examples of each type of poisoning. Place these examples and methods on a flip chart or chalkboard.
2. Ask participants to relate how different body systems are affected by different methods of poisoning.

Color Transparency 46

Flip Chart/ Chalkboard

Signals of Poisoning

Primary Points:

- Often the scene itself is the best clue that poisoning may have occurred. Factors to notice include—
    - Odors.
    - Flames or smoke.
    - Containers that are open or out-of-place.
    - Plants partially eaten or disturbed.
- Other signals of poisoning are common to all sudden illnesses, such as—
    - Nausea or vomiting.
    - Chest or abdominal pain.
    - Breathing difficulty.
    - Altered consciousness.
    - Seizures.
- Sometimes burns will be present on or around the mouth.

Transparency Master 48

Caring for Poisoning

Primary Points:

- The most important point is to call professional help if you suspect a poisoning.
- For conscious victims, call your closest Poison Control Center (PCC). (Give the number of the PCC center that serves your community.) If the victim is unconscious or you do not know the PCC number, call your local emergency number (e.g., 9–1–1).
- In addition, follow these basic steps:
  - Survey the scene to make sure it is safe.
  - Remove victim from the source of poison.
  - Do a primary survey.
  - Care for life-threatening conditions (such as absence of breathing) until professional help arrives.
  - Follow any advice from PCC given over the phone.
- You may be told to induce vomiting or to dilute the poison. Ask participants for examples of situations in which PCC may direct you to do either.

Color Transparency 47

Preventing Poisoning

Primary Points:

- Keep household products and medications out of the reach of children.
- Keep products in original containers.
- Use symbols to identify dangerous substances.
- Dispose of out-of-date products.
- Work with chemicals only in well-ventilated areas and with proper safety equipment and clothing.
- Educate others who may come in contact with poisonous substances about precautions they could take at work, home, or play.

Activity:

1. Summarize the lesson by having participants state some common signals of specific sudden illnesses such as fainting, diabetic emergencies, seizure, poisoning,

and stroke. Place participants' responses on one half of chalkboard or flip chart.

Flip Chart/ Chalkboard

2. Have participants offer steps of care for each sudden illness identified above. Place these steps on the other half of the flip chart or chalkboard.
3. Ask participants if they notice the similarities among illnesses. Reinforce that this is why participants do not have to "diagnose" problems. It is almost impossible to determine the exact cause, but **all** can be serious situations. Therefore, the cause does not matter, since all are cared for in the same basic manner: primary survey, calling EMS for professional help, and secondary survey when appropriate.

Transparency Master 49

Assignment:

- Read Chapter 15.
- Complete the Values Clarification Exercise in Chapter 15, page 328.

Lesson 25: SUBSTANCE MISUSE AND ABUSE

Class assignment prior to this lesson: Read Chapter 15. Complete the Values Clarification Exercise.

Length: 45 minutes

Needed: Textbook; transparency masters 50 and 51

Goal Statement: Participants should become familiar with the signals of substance misuse and abuse; general steps for providing care, and prevention strategies.

OVERVIEW SUBSTANCE MISUSE AND ABUSE

Instructor Notes

Time: 15 minutes

Note: You might invite the local drug enforcement agency (DEA) or police department's narcotics/vice, or community education groups to enhance discussions and identify specific drug problems in the participants' community.

Primary Points:

- Explain that substance misuse and abuse is actually poisoning of the body. Briefly review the methods of poisoning.
- Distinguish between substance misuse and substance abuse. Ask participants to give examples of each.

Activity:

1. Discuss the three general classifications of misused and abused substances. Explain that some substances do not fit well into any category (for example, "designer drugs").
2. Ask participants to identify possible physical and mental problems that are associated with misuse and abuse of different substances.
3. Read the following scenarios aloud to the class. Ask participants whether they feel each scenario indicates substance abuse or misuse.

Scenario 1
Alberta is a housewife with two young children. When she gets up in the morning, she must have her coffee and cigarettes. Throughout the day she smokes one pack of cigarettes and has six cups of coffee. She always has an after-dinner drink.

Scenario 2
Mike is a 21-year-old college student. On weekends, he goes to parties with his friends and drinks 8 to 10 beers from 9:00 p.m. to 1:00 a.m. The next morning he has difficulty getting up, feels nauseated, and has a headache.

Scenario 3
James is a 42-year-old construction worker, married, with children. Every day after work, he stops by a local pub and has three mixed drinks with his co-workers. He drives home and then has two more drinks with his dinner. He becomes very impatient and easily angered when his children play in the same room.

Scenario 4
Denise, age 22, goes to a social gathering at a co-worker's home. Throughout the evening, she drinks approximately six cocktails and eats very few of the hors d'oeuvres. Denise's speech starts slurring and she becomes unsteady. Her boyfriend makes an excuse for her behavior, and they leave the party. This is not the first time this has happened to Denise.

Scenario 5
Megan, age 17, severely sprains her ankle while playing soccer. When she goes home from practice, she is in a great deal of pain. She goes to the medicine cabinet and takes two pain pills that were prescribed when she had her wisdom teeth removed. She continues taking the pills over the next 48 hours.

Scenario 6
Stanley, a high school senior, has a 3.5 grade point average. He is looking forward to going to college and majoring in accounting. He smokes one marijuana cigarette, alone, every evening after studying. On weekends with his friends, he smokes several marijuana cigarettes while consuming alcohol.

Scenario 7
Maria, a recent college graduate, is teaching in an elementary school. She was overweight and consulted a physician about her diet. Her physician prescribed diet pills. Now she is at her goal weight but continues to take the diet pills to prevent a weight gain. The diet pill prescription has two remaining refills; she gets them filled. Even though she has already taken her prescribed daily dose, Maria takes a few more after an exhausting day at work. She claims they give her more energy.

FACTORS LEADING TO SUBSTANCE MISUSE AND ABUSE

Time: 10 minutes

Primary Points:

- Explain to participants that preventing substance misuse and abuse is an extremely complex process, not yet well understood or carried out.

Activity:

1. Review with participants the factors identified in the text as those that can lead to substance misuse and abuse.
2. Ask participants to give examples of how each of the problems identified in Activity 1 is or can lead to misuse and abuse.
3. Review with participants the five items identified in the textbook as bearing on individual decisions to use substances.

Textbook Transparency Master 50

4. Ask participants if they agree or disagree with each of the items and for examples of how these points have an impact on decisions to use substances.

INITIAL CARE FOR MISUSE AND ABUSE

Time: 10 minutes

Primary Points:

- Explain that signals of misuse and abuse can be similar to those of other medical emergencies.

Activity:

Ask the participants to list the general steps of care that may be needed for someone who misuses or abuses a substance. Use the following scenario to begin discussion of the primary point above.

Transparency Master 51

A 25-year-old woman has several drinks at a party. She later says that she feels dizzy and nauseated. She goes into another room. Soon after, someone enters shouting that she has collapsed to the floor and is unconscious. Among the objects scattered on the floor from her open purse are several containers of pills. One is marked "Valium." How would you help the woman? In terms of providing initial care, does it matter that she may have become unconscious because of substance misuse or abuse?

Note: The general care steps are the same for this scenario as for any medical emergency. The woman is unconscious. She needs to have the airway maintained and breathing and pulse checked. EMS personnel need to be summoned immediately. You cannot be certain that her problem is related to substance use.

PREVENTING MISUSE AND ABUSE

Time: 10 minutes

Primary Points:

- Explain that, once a decision has been made to use substances, it is difficult to change, since use becomes a habit.

Activity:

1. Either in small groups or as a single large group, begin discussion of the Values Clarification Exercise in the textbook. **Textbook**

   Note: Remember that there are no right or wrong responses because individuals' values differ. You might list responses to items such as "the greatest fear I would have about seeking help for a substance abuse problem..."

2. Summarize the lesson, emphasizing—
   - General classifications of substances.
   - Basic steps for care of substance-related emergencies.
   - That substance abuse and misuse is a very serious problem worldwide.
   - That participants should reevaluate their Healthy Lifestyles Awareness Inventory in light of what they learned and expressed in this lesson.

Assignment:

- Read Chapter 16.

Lesson 26: HEAT AND COLD EXPOSURE

Class assignment prior to this lesson: Read Chapter 16.

Length: 45 minutes

Needed: Color transparency 48; transparency masters 26, 52 through 60; self-assessment exercise 3

Goal Statement: Participants should become familiar with the signals of illness caused by heat or cold exposure, how to provide care, and prevention strategies.

REGULATING BODY TEMPERATURE

Instructor Notes

Time: 5 minutes

Overview

Primary Points:

- The body generates heat by converting food to energy and through muscle contractions.
- Normal body temperature is 98.6°F.
- Heat moves from warm areas (body core) to cooler areas (skin surface). This process helps maintains normal body temperature.
- When the body gets too hot, excessive heat is removed when blood vessels near the skin dilate. — **Color Transparency 48**
- When the body is cold, the opposite occurs. Blood vessels near the skin constrict, keeping warm blood in the center of the body.
- Sometimes constriction of blood vessels is not enough to keep the body warm. In this case, the body starts to shiver. Shivering produces heat through muscle action.

Factors Affecting Temperature Regulation

Primary Points:

- Factors affecting how well the body maintains normal temperature include— — **Transparency Master 52**
  - Air temperature.
  - Humidity.

- Wind.
- Clothing.
- Intensity of activity.
- Fluid intake.
- Adaptability of the body.

◆ Those at greatest risk of heat- or cold-related illnesses include—
- Young children.
- The elderly.
- Those involved in strenuous activity in a hot environment.
- Those with predisposing health problems.

Transparency Master 53

HEAT EMERGENCIES

Time: 10 minutes

Overview

Primary Points:

◆ Three conditions are associated with overexposure to heat: heat stroke, heat exhaustion, and heat cramps.

Transparency Master 54

◆ Heat cramps occur as a result of loss of both fluid and salt due to heavy sweating. They occur rapidly and involve painful spasms of skeletal muscles.

◆ A more serious heat-related condition, heat exhaustion, typically occurs after long periods of strenuous activity in a hot environment.

◆ Those often affected include—
- Athletes.
- Firefighters.
- Construction/factory workers.

◆ Heat exhaustion is an early indicator that the body's temperature-regulating mechanism is being overwhelmed.

◆ As the blood flow to the skin increases in an effort to remove heat from the body core, blood flow to vital organs is reduced. This results in a mild form of shock. Consequently, the shocklike signals present include—
- Dizziness/weakness.
- Cool, moist skin.
- Nausea.

- Heat stroke is the most severe of the heat-related emergencies. It occurs when the body is so overwhelmed by its high temperature that it fails to function properly.
- A series of life-threatening conditions occur:
  - Sweating stops as a result of low body fluid levels.
  - Body temperature rises rapidly, as a result of the lack of sweating.
  - The brain and other vital organs cannot function properly under excessive heat.
  - Unconsciousness and convulsions will occur.
  - Death can follow if the situation is not corrected rapidly.

Primary Points:

Caring for Heat Emergencies

Transparency Master 55

- The most important steps you can take for someone suspected of developing a heat-related emergency is to cool the victim's body and call EMS personnel.
- Cooling the body can be done by—
  - Removing the victim from the hot environment.
  - Giving small amounts of cool water to a conscious victim.
  - Loosening or removing clothing.
  - Applying cool, wet towels or sheets or cold packs to the body.
  - Fanning the victim.

COLD EMERGENCIES

Time: 10 minutes

Frostbite

Primary Points:

Transparency Master 56

- Frostbite is the actual freezing of body tissues. Body cells are damaged or destroyed when fluid in the cells freezes and swells.

- Factors affecting the extent of damage include—
  - Air temperature.
  - Wind speed.
  - Length of exposure.
  - Amount of exposed area.
- Frostbite can be either superficial or deep. Superficial frostbite is most common, occurring when the skin is frozen but the tissues below are not. Deep frostbite involves the freezing of both the skin and tissues below.
- Signals of frostbite include—
  - Skin that is cold to the touch.
  - Discolored skin (flushed, white, yellow, blue—depends on length of time without care after frostbite occurs).

Caring for Frostbite

Primary Points:

- Caring for frostbite involves the following:
  - Handle the affected area gently.
  - **Do not** rub the area.
  - Warm the affected area in water 100° to 105°F. This is the approximate temperature of a hot tub.
  - Once the affected area feels warm and appears red, remove it from the water and bandage loosely with dry materials.

Hypothermia

Primary Points:

- Unlike frostbite, which affects specific areas, hypothermia is the general cooling of the entire body.
- A growing concern in America is the number of people dying each year from cold exposure. These fatalities are associated with the growing homeless and older adult populations.
- Signals of hypothermia include—
  - Shivering (first response of the body to create heat through muscle contractions).

- Numbness.
- Apathy.
- Decreasing level of consciousness.

Caring for Hypothermia

Primary Points:

- ◆ To care for hypothermia, call EMS and rewarm the victim. This is done by—
  - Removing wet clothing.
  - Placing the victim in dry blankets or clothing.
  - Moving the victim to a warm environment.
  - Giving warm liquids to drink, if the victim is conscious.
  - Rewarming gradually.

PREVENTING HEAT AND COLD EMERGENCIES

Time: 10 minutes

Primary Points:

- ◆ Emergencies resulting from overexposure to extreme temperatures are preventable.

Activity:

1. Give the following scenario to the participants.

Transparency Master 57

Scenario

Twenty-year-old Todd Wilson is working for his uncle, remodeling, during the summer. He is putting fiberglass insulation in an attic. He is wearing long pants, a long-sleeved shirt, goggles, a face mask, and a hat to protect himself from contact with the irritating fiberglass.

Outdoor temperatures have been running about 90°F, and this day is exceptionally humid as well. Todd had hoped to have finished this job the evening before, but was unable to get to it until noon. He expects that it will take about 4½ hours.

Because Todd is in a hurry, he is working quickly to complete the job. He thinks that he may be able to save some time if he does not take any breaks. About two hours later, drenched with sweat, Todd starts to feel dizzy, weak, and nauseated. He barely has the energy to get down from the attic.

2. Ask participants to identify ways that the victim could have prevented this heat-related emergency.

   Note: Participant responses should include the following:
   - *Do not work in the hottest part of the day.*
   - *Take frequent breaks in cooler areas.*
   - *Drink large amounts of fluid.*
   - *Reduce the intensity of the work.*
   - *When possible, remove heavy clothing to cool down.*

YOU ARE THE CITIZEN RESPONDER

Time: 10 minutes

Activity:

1. Divide the participants into small groups. Give each group one of the "Putting It All Together" scenarios. (See pages 157 through 159 in this manual.)
2. Tell the participants they will be given 10 minutes to determine how best to respond to the emergency situation they have been given.
3. Remind the participants that they should use the Emergency Action Principles to guide their response.
4. Explain to participants that each group will present their scenario during the next lesson.
5. Distribute the 20– to 25–question self-assessment exercise 3 that you create from test bank questions. Explain to participants that they will review the exercise during the next lesson.

Transparency Master 26

Assignment:

- Review Chapters 13 through 16 and complete unanswered Study Questions.
- Complete self-assessment exercise 3.

Putting It All Together: Scenarios

Scenario 1
Sudden Illness

Transparency Master 58

For several hours, your 60-year-old uncle has been complaining of indigestion while at your home for a seafood cookout. He now states that he has severe stomach pain and is nauseated. He attributes this pain and nausea to the food he ate. You notice that his skin is rather pale, he is breathing rapidly, and he looks ill. You want to help. How do you proceed?

Note: Though participants might be thinking about food poisoning, there is no way to determine exactly what is wrong with the victim. However, it is unlikely that he is just having indigestion. The signals suggest that something more serious is wrong and that things are getting worse. He should stop any activity and rest in the most comfortable position. EMS personnel should be called, normal body temperature should be maintained, and ABCs monitored.

Scenario 2
Sudden Illness

An elderly neighbor is walking in front of your home. You notice him lose his balance and collapse to the ground. He is not fully conscious. His eyes are open, and the left side of his face appears to be drooping. The victim is making mumbling sounds, but you cannot tell what he is saying. Suddenly, he begins to vomit. You want to help. How do you proceed?

Note: It is possible that this person is experiencing a stroke. However, the care for this person should be based on the signals present, rather than on an ability to "diagnose" the underlying problem.

If he is not already on his side, the victim should be rolled over so that the vomitus can drain from his mouth. The priority here is to keep the airway clear. The responder should shout for help to attract any neighbors.

If someone arrives, he or she should be told to call EMS personnel and then return to help provide care. Continue to monitor the ABCs until professional help arrives. Scan the body to make sure that no severe bleeding has resulted from the fall. There is no need to do a secondary survey, since your priorities involve the ABCs. If the man stops breathing, rescue breathing should be done.

Scenario 3
Heat-Related Emergency

Transparency Master 59

It is late in the afternoon, and your team is finishing its third match of the volleyball tournament on the beach. It has been a really hot day, with temperatures in the 90s. Suddenly, a teammate collapses. She does not appear to be fully conscious, but is breathing rapidly. You notice that her skin is very warm, sunburned, and moist. Her pulse is very fast. She is unable to get up from the ground. You want to help. How do you proceed?

Note: Given the fact that the victim has been involved in a great deal of strenuous activity in a hot environment, it is possible that she is suffering from heat-related illness. The physical signals also suggest this possibility. She should be removed from the heat as quickly as possible. This might involve lifting and moving her, either alone or with the help of teammates. She should be taken to a shaded area, air-conditioned building, shower area, or air-conditioned vehicle. If none of these are available nearby, she could be moved to the cool, wet sand near the water and shaded from direct sunlight. If lifeguards are nearby, get them to assist. EMS personnel should be called. Try to cool the victim, using wet towels, sheets, or blankets. Since she is not fully conscious, do not give any fluids. She should be placed flat on her back, and her ABCs monitored until EMS personnel arrive.

Scenario 4
Substance Abuse

Transparency Master 60

A dangerous ritual is about to begin—21 drinks for the 21st birthday. A group of close friends has gathered for a special party for the "birthday boy." Everyone knows it is a dangerous game, but, because each of these friends went through it, they believe it is a rite of passage into adulthood. The activities begin, and the guest of honor is soon "chugging beers" and downing shots of liquor at a rapid pace. Two hours after the drinking began, you arrive at the party. The guest of honor is vomiting violently in the bathroom. He slumps to the floor and begins violent convulsions, followed by unconsciousness. He seems to stop breathing and then takes a deep breath. You are summoned to help. How do you proceed?

Note: It is clear that the victim is experiencing alcohol poisoning. His airway should be cleared, ABCs monitored, and EMS personnel called immediately. If possible, he should be removed from the bathroom to a more open area with additional space, making it easier to work with him. If he stops breathing, give rescue breathing. Monitor pulse periodically to be certain he still has a heartbeat.

Lesson 27: PUTTING IT ALL TOGETHER

Class assignment prior to this lesson:	Review Chapters 13 through 16 and complete unanswered Study Questions. Complete self-assessment exercise 3.
Length:	45 minutes
Needed:	Transparency masters 26, 58 through 60; blankets or mats; manikins (optional); decontamination supplies; self-assessment 3 answer key
Goal Statement:	Given a series of medical emergencies, participants should be able to make appropriate decisions regarding care and demonstrate proper first aid techniques.

YOU ARE THE CITIZEN RESPONDER

Time: 35 minutes

Activity:

1. Divide the participants into their small groups from the previous lesson. Give each group a few minutes to review the plan of action for their "Putting It All Together" scenario.

   Note: Remind participants that they are expected to be able to discuss or demonstrate any previously learned skill that is required to respond effectively. If the group feels it is necessary to use a skill they have not learned (such as movement of a victim from a dangerous area), they may simply verbalize their actions and will not be required to demonstrate the skill.

2. Remind the participants that they should use the Emergency Action Principles to guide their responses.
3. One at a time, use the transparency or have participants read the scenario aloud to the class and role-play their response to the emergency. Tell the participants that they should demonstrate any previously learned skill that would be required as an effective response.

   At any time during the role-play, they may choose to use either a manikin or a

Instructor Notes

Blankets or Mats

Manikins (optional)

Decontamination Supplies

Transparency Masters 58 through 60

member of the group as the victim. Each group should discuss their actions while giving care. They should also be able to answer questions the instructor or other participants may have.

4. After a group has role-played a specific scenario, initiate a discussion by asking the class to evaluate the group's response, using the questions below. Each scenario and accompanying discussion should take about seven minutes.

Plan of Action

- Did the group's plan follow the Emergency Action Principles?
  - Survey the scene
  - Primary survey
  - Call EMS
  - Secondary survey
- Did the plan involve bystanders appropriately?
- Did the plan demonstrate proper care?
- In addition, ask what specific signals the group noticed that may have suggested the type of medical emergency they encountered.

Transparency Master 26

5. At the end of this activity, answer any questions that participants may have. Make sure that all participants have an opportunity to resolve their confusions or have their questions answered.

REVIEW SELF-ASSESSMENT EXERCISE

Time: 10 minutes

Self-Assessment Exercise 3

Activity:

Self-assessment 3 answer key

1. Ask the participants to get out their completed self-assessment exercises.
2. Ask each participant to read aloud one question and its answer. Have participants include a very brief reason for why they think the answer is correct. Explain

that participants can ask the class for help if they do not know the answer to a particular question.

3. Proceed sequentially through each of the questions until all have been answered.

Assignment:

- Read Chapter 17.

Lesson 28: RESCUE MOVES

Class assignment prior to this lesson: Read Chapter 17.

Length: 45 minutes

Needed: Video; transparency masters 26, 61 through 65; flip chart or chalkboard

Goal Statement: Participants will become familiar with methods of assisting people in dangerous situations.

LAND RESCUE

Time: 15 minutes

Instructor Notes

Overview

Primary Points:

- Sometimes a victim must be rescued from a dangerous situation before care can be given.
- There are several methods of moving a victim that can be done simply and with little danger of injury to you or the victim.

Moving Victims

Primary Points:

- To protect yourself and the victim from injury, follow these basic guidelines:
  - Move only a victim you can comfortably handle.
  - Bend at your knees.
  - Lift with your legs, not your back.
  - Take short steps.
  - Move forward whenever possible.
  - Look where you are walking.
  - Protect against head and spine injury.

Transparency Master 61

- There are limitations to every rescue situation. To move one or more victims quickly and safely, participants should evaluate these limitations. Evaluate—
  - The extent of the danger at the scene.
  - The size of victim(s).
  - The physical ability of rescuer(s).
  - Whether others can help.
  - The victim's condition.

Transparency Master 62

- Explain to participants that they are about to watch a video demonstrating several common types of emergency moves.

  Note: If you choose not to show this video segment, demonstrate five emergency moves discussed in the textbook. Show techniques to prevent back injury to the rescuer. Ensure that all participants can see the demonstration.

Video: Show the final video segment: *Rescue Moves* (03:00).

Activity:

1. Ask participants to recall the common types of emergency moves. List them on flip chart or chalkboard.
2. Ask participants to give an example of a situation in which each type of move is appropriate as well as any limitation inherent in the move. (For example, a fireman's carry is not good for possible head, spine, or abdominal injury.) List them next to the emergency moves.
3. Answer any questions that participants may have regarding proper movement of a victim on land.

Flip Chart/ Chalkboard

WATER RESCUE

Time: 15 minutes

Drowning

Primary Points:

- Drowning is death by suffocation when submerged in water.
- Near-drowning refers to a victim surviving submersion (although sometimes only temporarily).

Assisting a Near-Drowning Victim

Note: Consider using a pool to demonstrate the assists mentioned here (or show the American Red Cross Emergency Aquatic Skills video (Stock No. 329331), which demonstrates these skills). If you do use a pool, recognize that this session will probably run longer than planned.

Primary Points:

- Do not endanger yourself in any water rescue.
- The safest methods are reaching, throwing, and wading assists.
- Reaching assists involve bracing yourself against the pool deck, ladder, or dock and extending your reach to a victim. You may use any device to extend your reach. You may also enter the water and hold on to a fixture, such as a pool ladder, while extending your reach.
- Throwing assists involve tossing a floatable object (either with or without a line attached) to a victim.
- When using a throwing assist, follow these guidelines:
    - Keep your balance. (Stand where you are safe.)
    - Secure any line that is being used to throw an object to a victim.
    - Throw the device beyond the victim.
    - Consider the wind or current when throwing a device.
    - Once the victim grasps the device, pull him or her slowly to safety if a line is attached.
    - If no line is attached, have the victim hold the device and kick to safety.
- If you choose to enter the water and wade out to the victim, be cautious of any sudden dropoff or current. Extend an object, such as a branch or pole, to the victim.

Survival Swimming

Primary Points:

- You may some day unexpectedly find yourself in the water while fully clothed. Try to float, either on your back or facedown. (Remember, facedown floating is not recommended for cold water.)
- Use your clothes to help make you more buoyant. A long-sleeved buttoned shirt

traps air well. Fasten all buttons except one in the middle of the shirt. Blow air into the shirt, and secure the button.

Primary Points:

Preventing Drowning

Transparency Master 63

- Most drownings happen to victims who never intended to enter the water.
- Take precautions such as—
  - Respecting the power of water.
  - Closely supervising children.
  - Wearing approved flotation devices when boating.
  - Swimming with a buddy in a supervised area.
  - Never using alcohol or other substances that would impair judgment or physical ability.

YOU ARE THE CITIZEN RESPONDER

Time: 15 minutes

Group Activity:

1. Present the scenarios one at a time to the class as a group. (See pages 169 through 170 in this manual).
2. Ask participants the following:
   - Would you move or rescue the victim?
   - If so, how would this be accomplished?
   - What care should the victim be given?

Transparency Master 26

3. Remind participants to use the Emergency Action Principles to guide their answers. The group's plan should follow these principles:
   - Survey the scene.
   - Primary survey.
   - Call EMS.
   - Secondary survey.

   The plan should also—
   - Involve bystanders appropriately.
   - Demonstrate proper care.
4. At the end of the lesson, answer any questions that participants still have. Make sure that the participants have an

opportunity to resolve their confusions by having questions answered.

Assignment:

- Read Chapter 18.
- Complete Healthy Lifestyles Awareness Inventory again.
- Bring textbook to class.

Scenarios

Scenario 1

Transparency Master 64

You are driving home with a friend at rush hour and witness an automobile collision involving one vehicle that has struck a guard rail head-on. The car is still running. The driver did not have on a safety belt and struck the steering column. He is seated behind the steering wheel, conscious and complaining of chest and abdominal pain. The other passenger also was not wearing a safety belt. She is lying motionless, facedown on the floor of the vehicle. You see blood around her body. She is unconscious and not breathing. You are unsure if she has a pulse. How do you proceed?

Note: You should take precautions such as using your vehicle and emergency flashers to slow any oncoming traffic. You should be cautious of any traffic as you walk toward the victims. You should attempt to flag down other motorists to help. If you can easily gain access to either side of the vehicle, you can assess the injuries to the victims. You do not need to move the driver of the vehicle. Stabilize the head in line with the body and monitor the ABCs. The passenger ***does*** *need to be moved, since rescue breathing may need to be done and you may need to make a better evaluation of whether or not a pulse is present. Bleeding must also be controlled. Other motorists can assist you in moving the victim as quickly as possible with the least movement of the victim. Other motorists can also be used to notify EMS personnel and assist with rescue breathing and CPR, if needed.*

Transparency Master 65

Scenario 2
There is a chemical explosion at an industrial plant. A worker nearby has been injured. She has severe burns on her face, neck, chest, and arms. She has walked into another room away from the explosion and collapsed to the floor. She is conscious with no other apparent injuries. There is danger of another explosion. You and a co-worker are close by and available to come to her aid. How do you proceed?

Note: If you decide to help her, the possibility of a second explosion makes it important for you to move her to safety. If protective masks are available, put one on to help prevent inhalation of poisonous substances before going to her aid. You might have to move the victim outside the building. You and your co-worker could use a two-person carry to move the victim to safety. Carry her away from the scene quickly, but carefully. Provide care for burns by cooling the burned areas. Monitor ABCs, minimize shock, and call EMS personnel.

Lesson 29: YOUR GUIDE TO A HEALTHIER LIFE

Class assignment prior to this lesson: Read Chapter 18. Complete the Healthy Lifestyles Awareness Inventory.

Length: 45 minutes

Needed: Textbook; transparency masters 66 through 68

Goal Statement: Participants will become familiar with various ways to lead a healthier life by preventing illness and injury.

LEADING A HEALTHY LIFESTYLE

Instructor Notes

Time: 5 minutes

Overview

Primary Points:

- The first aid knowledge you have gained in this course is essential to dealing with emergencies promptly and effectively. However, this knowledge does not help you **prevent** the emergency from occurring in the first place.
- Preventing illness or injury is the most important aspect of leading a healthy lifestyle. It is far more effective to prevent illness or injury than to provide care for it once it happens.
- A healthy lifestyle is a combination of positive beliefs and practices that help form good habits in many areas of your life, which can help prevent injury or illness.
- These good habits involve areas such as proper nutrition, exercise, and safety.
- Your present and future health and well-being depend on preventing injury or illness.

CARING FOR YOUR BODY

Time: 25 minutes

Nutrition

Primary Points:

◆ Proper nutrition means eating a balanced diet. This is done by balancing foods from the four basic food groups:
- Carbohydrates
- Dairy products
- Proteins
- Fruit and vegetables

Transparency Master 66

Activity:

Ask participants to name at least four examples of foods that fit into each of these four basic food groups.

Weight

Primary Points:

◆ Maintaining appropriate body weight will help reduce your chances of illness.

◆ The presence of too much fat is of greatest concern when evaluating body weight because it contributes to disease.

◆ Physicians or health care specialists, such as those found at fitness centers, can help you identify your appropriate body weight by measuring your percentage of body fat.

Note: If you are knowledgeable about techniques used to determine body fat measurements and have access to the necessary equipment, you might want to demonstrate how these measurements are frequently taken.

◆ Your eating habits should be adjusted as you age. Because your metabolism slows down, you will tend to gain weight if your eating habits and activity level remain constant.

Exercise

Primary Points:

◆ Any attempts to gain or lose weight should be accompanied by regular exercise.

- Exercise is good for the heart, lungs, and blood vessels. It increases endurance, strength, and flexibility.
- The foundation of whole-body fitness lies with cardiovascular fitness. Cardiovascular fitness helps you—

  Transparency Master 67

  - Cope with stress.
  - Control weight.
  - Fight off infections.
  - Improve self-esteem.
  - Sleep better.
- Achieving cardiovascular fitness means exercising your heart. You should exercise three times a week, for approximately 30 minutes each time, and at your Target Heart Rate.
- Target Heart Rate is 65 to 80 percent of maximum heart rate. Determining Target Heart Rate involves using a formula. By using the following formula, you can determine your own Target Heart Rate: 220 – Age ***x*** (.65 to .80) = Target Heart Rate; (i.e.) 220 – 20 ***x*** .65 = 130 beats per minute; (i.e.) 220 – 20 ***x*** .80 = 160 beats per minute
- Given the above examples, a 20-year-old person should get his or her heart rate up to between 130 and 160 beats per minute and keep it in this range for approximately 30 minutes. This should be done three times a week.

Activity: Have participants determine their own Target Heart Rate using the same formula.

Controlling Stress

Primary Points:

- Handling stress successfully often requires that you direct your attention to something—such as enjoyable hobbies—other than what is causing the stress. For some people, this involves physical activities. For others, relaxation exercises help the body to relax.

Note: If your environment is conducive to practicing relaxation exercises, follow these basic guidelines to enable participants to experience stress reduction. Otherwise, present these as primary points.

Activity:

1. Have participants get as comfortable as possible. This could be either sitting or lying down.
2. Dim the lights in the classroom.
3. Have participants close their eyes.
4. Ask participants to focus on their breathing. Breathe in deeply through the nose, and exhale through the mouth. Do this for five-to-ten minutes.

   Note: Other techniques that can help include playing soft music in the background, having participants tighten and then relax muscles throughout the body, and listening to the sound of a soft voice guiding participants through the exercise.

Breaking Unhealthy Habits

Primary Points:

- Cigarette smoking is a habit that brings with it some very unhealthy consequences—increased risks of heart disease and cancer.
- Consuming alcohol in large amounts can affect the body in adverse ways. It—
  - Impairs judgment.
  - Slows reflexes.
  - Makes driving unsafe.
  - Can result in disease if consumption is prolonged.
- When hosting a party (or being a party participant), basic guidelines to follow include—
  - Drinking no more than one drink per hour.
  - Having nonalcoholic beverages available.
  - Avoiding drinking if depressed or angry.

Transparency Master 68

- Not drinking before a party.
- Having plenty of food available.
- Avoiding drinking games.
- Having designated drivers.

Medical and Dental Care

Primary Points:

- ◆ Regular medical and dental checkups will help you prevent disease.
- ◆ Age, personal and family history, and other factors have an impact on how frequently you need medical exams.
- ◆ Have dental checkups twice a year.

Preventing Injury

Primary Points:

- ◆ Injuries are a leading cause of death and disability in the United States.
- ◆ Following fire-safety tips can prevent many fire-related incidents.
- ◆ If a fire does break out, you should have a well-rehearsed fire evacuation plan.
- ◆ Whether at home or work, take steps to keep your environment safe.

Activity:

Ask participants to identify ways to keep their home and work area safe. List the ways they suggest. The list should include—

- ◆ Posting emergency numbers.
- ◆ Maintaining proper lighting.
- ◆ Using handrails.
- ◆ Maintaining heating and cooling systems.
- ◆ Following manufacturer's instructions when using equipment or appliances.
- ◆ Unplugging potential fire-causing items.
- ◆ Keeping a fire extinguisher in an accessible area.
- ◆ Locking up poisonous substances and firearms.
- ◆ Having an emergency action plan in case of illness or injury.

REVIEWING THE HEALTHY LIFESTYLES AWARENESS INVENTORY

Time: 15 minutes

Healthy Lifestyles Awareness Inventory

Activity:

After the participants have completed the Healthy Lifestyles Awareness Inventory as assigned, ask them to tally their scores, if they have not already done so. Have the participants record their scores on the Score Card II (Appendix D, textbook), and turn it in to you. Tell participants that it is not necessary for them to put their names on the score card.

Note: The purpose of having you receive all of the participants' scores is to tally the total class score to compute the class average. By comparing it with the average calculated at the beginning of the course, you can determine if there is any improvement in group behavior.

Self-Evaluation

Activity:

1. Ask the participants to divide into small groups (three or four) to discuss the results of each participant's inventory, identifying areas in which improvement was made, or in which it is still needed.
2. Ask participants to discuss their findings and reflect on the Behavior Modification Contracts they completed at the start of the course (if they did this).
3. Compute the scores and provide the participants with feedback regarding the comparison of class average between the start of the course and now.
4. Note any significant findings.
5. Answer any questions participants may have.

Assignment:

- Ask participants to begin reviewing all chapters, and completing unanswered study questions, for the upcoming review and final written examination.

Lesson 30: PUTTING IT ALL TOGETHER: REVIEWING THE COURSE

Class assignment prior to this lesson: Begin reviewing chapters and completing any unanswered study questions.

Length: 45 minutes

Needed: Transparency masters 69 and 70; blankets or mats; bandaging and splinting equipment or supplies; manikins (optional); decontamination supplies

Goal Statement: This lesson is designed to provide participants an opportunity for a comprehensive self-assessment of the knowledge and skills acquired throughout this course.

Given a series of scenarios involving life-threatening and non-life-threatening situations, participants will be able to make appropriate decisions for care and demonstrate proper first aid techniques.

YOU ARE THE CITIZEN RESPONDER

Time: 45 minutes

Activity:

1. Explain to participants that this lesson will give them an opportunity to review major points learned in this course.
2. Explain that they will be presented with various scenarios to which they are expected to respond.
3. Explain to participants that, as they respond, you will provide them with verbal prompts and information.

Note: The scenarios are on pages 178 through 189 in this manual. Structure them in any manner desirable to accomplish the goal of reviewing the course with the participants. You may want to present these scenarios in small groups, or to the class as a whole. Involve as many participants as possible in the scenarios.

Instructor Notes

Blankets or Mats

Bandaging and Splinting Equipment

Manikins (optional)

Decontamination Supplies

Putting It All Together: Reviewing the Course

Instructor Notes

Primary Points:

- Remind the participants that a basic plan of action was followed in all the scenarios. It included—
  - Survey the scene.
  - Primary survey.
  - Call EMS.
  - Secondary survey.
- Explain to participants that they have just reviewed the major segments of the course. They have successfully reviewed proper care for—
  - Airway obstruction.
  - Respiratory arrest.
  - Cardiac arrest.
  - Severe bleeding.
  - Musculoskeletal injuries.
  - Medical emergencies: unconsciousness, seizures, diabetic emergencies.
- In the time remaining, answer any questions participants may have.

Assignment:

- Review Chapters 1 through 18 and Study Questions for the final written examination.

Scenarios

Scenario 1

Transparency Master 69

As you are being escorted to your table in a restaurant, a man hastens by you, coughing repeatedly. A few minutes later, the maitre d' rushes in, asking for assistance. You overhear him, and decide to help. As you are led outside, you see a man lying facedown on the sidewalk, not moving. Others have gathered around, but no one is doing anything. You recognize the man as the one who rushed past you in the restaurant. How do you proceed?

Note: What follows is a progression of appropriate participant actions, and instructor prompts. Participant actions may vary somewhat from the order presented on the following page.

Segment 1A	
Participant Actions	**Instructor Prompts**
1. **Survey the scene.** (Look around to see that it is safe.)	**"Scene is safe."**
2. **Ask initial questions.** (Does anyone know what hap-pened?)	**"He appeared to be choking, collapsed to his knees, then passed out."**
3. **Check consciousness.** (Tap and shout.)	**"There is no response."**
4. **Recruit help.** (Ask bystanders to assist you.)	**"Two people kneel down to help you."**
5. **Position victim.** (Roll victim onto back.)	**"Victim on back."**
6. **Open airway.** (Head-tilt/chin-lift.)	**"Airway appears open."**
7. **Check for breathing**. (Look, listen, and feel.)	**"Victim is not breathing."**
8. **Give 2 breaths.** (Look for chest rise.)	**"Breaths do not go in."**
9. **Reposition head**. (Retilt head and lift chin.)	**"Head is repositioned."**
10. **Repeat breaths**. (Look for chest rise.)	**"Breaths still do not go in."**
11. **Notify EMS personnel.** (Send bystander with information.)	**"Bystander calls EMS."**

Segment 1A (con't.)	
Participant Actions	**Instructor Prompts**
12. **Give 6 to 10 abdominal thrusts**. (Below xiphoid, above navel.)	**"Good thrusts."**
13. **Perform finger sweep.** (Lift jaw, use hooking action.)	**"No object found."**
14. **Open airway.** (Head-tilt/chin-lift.)	**"Airway appears open."**
15. **Attempt 2 breaths**.	**"Breaths still do not go in."**
16. **Repeat abdominal thrusts.**	**"Good thrusts."**
17. **Repeat finger sweep**.	**"Object removed."**

* * * **STOP** * * *

(At this point, consider having others continue the scenario.)

Segment 1B	
The victim did have an airway obstruction, and the object has now been removed. How do you continue to provide care?	
Participant Actions	**Instructor Prompts**
18. **Open the airway**. (Head-tilt/chin-lift.)	**"Airway appears open."**
19. **Check for breathing**. (Look, listen, feel.)	**"Victim is still not breathing."**
20. **Give 2 breaths**. (Look for chest rise.)	**"Breaths go in."**
21. **Check circulation**. (Check pulse, severe bleeding.)	**"No pulse. — No bleeding evident."**
22. **Give 15 chest compressions.**	**"Good compressions."**
23. **Give 2 breaths.**	**"Breaths go in."**
24. **Repeat 3 cycles of CPR.**	**"One minute of CPR has been done."**
25. **Recheck pulse**.	**"Pulse present."**

* * * **STOP** * * *

(At this point, consider having others continue the scenario.)

Segment 1C	
The victim now has a pulse. How do you continue to provide care?	
Participant Actions	**Instructor Prompts**
26. **Recheck breathing.** (Look, listen, feel.)	**"Victim is still not breathing."**
27. **Do rescue breathing.** (1 breath every 5 seconds.)	**After about 30 seconds: "Victim vomits."**
28. **Roll victim onto side.** (Use bystanders if possible.)	**"Victim is still vomiting."**
29. **Clear the airway.** (Sweep mouth clear using finger.)	**"Airway appears clear."**
30. **Reposition victim on back.**	**"Victim on back."**
31. **Open airway.** (Head-tilt/chin-lift.)	**"Airway appears open."**
32. **Check breathing.** (Look, listen, feel.)	**"Victim is now breathing but still unconscious."**

* * * **STOP** * * *

(At this point, consider having others continue the scenario.)

The victim is now breathing. What further care should be provided until EMS personnel arrive?

- ◆ Maintain an open airway.
- ◆ Monitor breathing and pulse.

- Maintain normal body temperature.
- Make sure EMS personnel have been called.

Answer any questions that participants may still have regarding the decisions made and care given.

Scenario 2

Your younger sister is taking riding lessons at a nearby ranch. You go with her one day to watch her practice. Today, she is riding a different horse from the one she normally rides. Suddenly, she is thrown from the horse. She falls flat on her back, striking her head on the ground. She lies motionless on the ground. The horse trots nearby. Her riding instructor is present to help. How do you proceed?

What follows is a progression of appropriate participant actions and instructor prompts. Participant actions may vary somewhat from the order of those presented below.

Segment 2A	
Participant Actions	**Instructor Prompts**
1. **Survey the scene.** (Have riding instructor secure horse.)	**"Scene is now safe."**
2. **Check consciousness.** (Tap and shout.)	**"There is no response."**
3. **Recruit help** (Shout to the riding instructor or others for help.)	**"Two people respond to your shouts."**

Segment 2A (con't.)	
Participant Actions	**Instructor Prompts**
4. **Limit further movement of the victim's head.** (Have a bystander use in-line stabilization.)	**"Head is stabilized."**
5. **Try to check breathing without moving the victim's head.** (Look, listen, feel.)	**"Victim is breathing."**
6. **Check circulation.** (Check for severe bleeding.)	**"No external bleeding present."**
7. **Notify EMS.** (Send bystander with information.)	**"Bystander calls EMS."**
8. **Monitor ABCs.**	**"ABCs being monitored."**

* * * **STOP** * * *

(At this point, consider having others continue the scenario.)

Segment 2B	
At this point, you have done all that you need to do. How would you continue to provide care if the victim's condition suddenly changed? What if the victim began having a seizure?	
Participant Actions	**Instructor Prompts**
9. **Protect the victim from further injury.** (Fold a shirt or sweater thinly, and place under the victim's head to limit further injury. Maintain in-line stabilization.)	**After pad is in place: "Seizure stops, but victim vomits."**
10. **Roll victim onto side.** (Use bystander to help roll victim.)	**"Victim is still vomiting."**
11. **Clear airway.** (Sweep mouth clear using finger.)	**"Airway appears clear."**
12. **Reposition victim on back.**	**"Victim is on back."**
13. **Try to check breathing without moving victim's head.** (Look, listen, feel.)	**"Victim is still breathing and begins to regain consciousness."**

* * * **STOP** * * *

(At this point, consider having others continue the scenario.)

The victim is breathing and regaining consciousness. Answer the following questions:

1. Should the victim be allowed to get up if she becomes conscious?
   - No. Care should continue to be provided for a possible serious head or spine injury. The victim should be encouraged to remain still.
2. What further care should be provided until EMS personnel arrive?
   - Monitor ABCs.
   - Maintain normal body temperature.
   - Make sure EMS personnel have been called.

* * * **STOP** * * *

Scenario 3

Transparency Master 70

You and your brother have just finished some yard work. Your brother goes inside to clean up. While still outside, you hear the sound of a chain saw nearby. You remember a neighbor saying that he was going to remove a large, dead tree in his yard. You decide to go over and see what is going on. Before you get far, you hear the sound of cracking wood, then you suddenly hear the saw stop, followed immediately by screams. You rush to your neighbor's yard. You see your neighbor sitting on the ground. Blood is pouring from a deep, large laceration just above his knee. Your neighbor is already "white as a ghost," is still screaming, and appears panic stricken. He is not making any effort to control the bleeding. You are alone with him. How do you proceed?

What follows is a progression of appropriate participant actions and instructor prompts. Participant actions may vary somewhat from the order presented on the following page.

Participant Actions	Instructor Prompts
1. **Survey the scene.** (Look around to see that the tree or branches are not about to fall.)	**"Scene is safe."**
2. **Shout for help**.	**"No one responds."**
3. **Check circulation.** (Look for severe bleeding.)	**"Severe bleeding is present."**
4. **Control bleeding**. (Use direct pressure and any barrier, such as clothing, over the wound. Ask victim to help.)	**"Victim is able to help you apply pressure."**
5. **Control bleeding.** (Elevate limb by placing nearby object under it.)	**"Limb is elevated."**
6. **Notify EMS personnel.** (Use neighbor's phone.)	**"EMS notified."**
7. **Recheck the bleeding**.	**"Blood is soaking through covering."**
8. **Control bleeding**. (Add more coverings. Apply pressure bandage by tearing clothing or using any supplies in the neighbor's home.)	**"Pressure bandage applied. Victim states he is dizzy and feels sick."**
9. **Minimize shock**. (Have victim lie down. Monitor ABCs. Maintain normal body temperature.)	**"Bleeding appears to be controlled. Victim states that he feels better."**

Bleeding has been controlled and shock minimized. What problem(s) did this rescuer have to overcome? How else might these problems have been overcome?

Problem	**Solution**
No one to help.	Possibly, call your own home to get help after calling EMS.
No equipment or supplies.	Modify any existing items for use.

*** * * STOP * * ***

Scenario 4

In the middle of a pick-up basketball game at a local playground, two players go up for a rebound. As they collide, they both lose their balance and fall to the ground. As one player lands, she twists her ankle violently. The other player falls on an outstretched arm and appears to have injured her wrist and forearm. Both victims are conscious and moaning. How do you proceed?

Participant Actions	**Instructor Prompts**
1. **Recruit help.** (Ask bystanders to help you.)	**"Several bystanders offer to help."**
2. **Do a secondary survey: interview.** (Ask about painful areas, ability to move, and sensation.)	**"Both injuries are painful, numb, and cannot be moved without further pain."**
3. **Do a secondary survey: check vital signs.** (Check pulse, respiration, skin.)	**"Vital signs are normal."**

Participant Actions	Instructor Prompts
4. **Do a secondary survey: head-to-toe examination.** (Rule out any other injuries. Check injury site for swelling, discoloration, cool feeling, bleeding, and so on.)	**"No other injuries present. Injury sites are both swollen, discolored, have normal temperature, and no external bleeding."**
5. **Immobilize injuries.** (Let ground splint ankle. Have someone stabilize it. Allow other victim to support arm against chest, or apply sling, binder and bind.)	**"Injuries are immobilized."**
6. **Notify EMS personnel.** (Send someone to call for help.)	**"EMS notified."**

* * * **STOP** * * *

You have successfully immobilized the injuries. What additional care could you provide?

- Minimize shock. Apply cold compress (if available). Help victims rest comfortably.

Lesson 31: FINAL WRITTEN EXAMINATION

Class assignment prior to this lesson: Review Chapters 1 through 18.

Length: 45 minutes

Needed: Final written examinations; answer sheets; answer key; participant course evaluations (Appendix D); pencils

Goal Statement: The purpose of this session is to evaluate how well participants understand the information that was presented in this course.

FINAL WRITTEN EXAMINATION

Time: 45 minutes

Instructor Notes

Activity:

1. Tell the participants that the written examination consists of 70 multiple-choice questions from the textbook for this course. Participants must answer at least 56 questions correctly in order to pass the examination. They may not use their textbook to find the answers.

Written examinations
Answer sheets
Pencils

2. Give an examination and answer sheet to each participant.
3. Briefly review the examination instructions that follow:
   - Instruct the participants to write only on the answer sheet.
   - All answers should be clearly marked.
   - Participants are encouraged to use a pencil to mark their answers in case they would like to erase or change their answers.
   - Tell participants to check their answers before handing them in.
4. Tell the participants they have approximately 35 minutes to complete the test. Some participants may need extra time to complete the exam. Try to be flexible to accommodate their needs.
5. Tell participants to come to you or to raise their hand when they have completed the examinations or have any specific questions.

Answer Key

6. Score the examinations. The answer keys for both examinations are in Appendix B.

   Note: Scoring keys are included at the end of this manual. If you place the appropriate scoring key over an answer sheet and align the corners of the answer sheet and the answer key, the correct answers will show through the punched holes. The passing grade for the written examination is 80 percent. (Participants must answer 56 out of 70 questions correctly.) For more information on course completion criteria, see Chapter 5, Requirements for Successful Course Completion, in this manual.

   As participants hand in their answer sheets, you may quickly grade the examination and return it to the participant so that he or she can review any missed questions. Collect all answer sheets and examinations before the participants leave the class. If a participant fails the examination, ask him or her to see you after class to schedule a retest.

   Refer to Chapter 6, "Course Conclusion" in Part A of this manual for information on what you need to do at the end of the course.

Participant Course Evaluations

7. Ask participants to complete the participant Course Evaluation (Appendix D). Give evaluations to all the participants as they complete the written examination, and ask them to leave the evaluations in a box or envelope you have provided near the door.
8. Thank all participants for attending the course.

Appendix A

Recommendations on Manikin Decontamination

Excerpted from "Standards and Guidelines for Cardiopulmonary Resuscitation and Emergency Cardiac Care," Journal of the American Medical Association *255, no. 21 (June 6, 1986): 2926–2928. Copyright 1986, American Medical Association. Used with permission.*

SAFETY IN TRAINING FOR AND PROVIDING CPR

Safety in CPR training from the students' and instructors' perspective has gained increased attention. Adherence to the following recommendations should minimize any possible complications for instructors and students during CPR training.

Disease Transmission and CPR Training
The following recommendations[67] for decontaminating manikins used in CPR training were updated in 1983 by members of the Multidisciplinary Ad Hoc Committee for Evaluation of Sanitary Practices in Cardiopulmonary Resuscitation Training. The committee was represented by the American Heart Association (Subcommittee on Emergency Cardiac Care), the American Red Cross (First Aid and CPR Programs), and the Centers for Disease Control (Center for Infectious Diseases and Laboratory Program Office). Instructors should follow these recommendations (which are directly quoted from the Centers for Disease Control) when manikins are used in CPR training.

In past years, we have received numerous inquiries concerning the possible role of cardiopulmonary resuscitation (CPR) training manikins in transmitting viral hepatitis type B. Recently, inquiries have been received about the potential for transmission of not only hepatitis B but also acquired immunodeficiency syndrome (AIDS), herpes viruses, and various upper and lower respiratory infections (influenza, infectious mononucleosis, tuberculosis, etc.). The use of CPR manikins has increased rapidly because of expanded training programs sponsored by medical and emergency organizations. To date, it is estimated that over 40 million people have had direct contact with manikins during training courses. In the United States, a number of companies distribute multiple model lines of manikins for training programs in hospitals, police and fire departments, service organizations, lay groups, and schools as part of health, first aid, and physical education courses. Since practicing with a manikin is an integral part of CPR training, the care and maintenance of the manikins is of utmost importance. Instructors and training agencies rely heavily on manufacturer's recommendations for manikin use and maintenance, and these recommendations for manikin use and maintenance should be examined carefully before purchasing manikins.

The use of CPR training manikins has never been documented as being responsible for an outbreak or even an isolated case of bacterial, fungal, or viral disease. However, manikin surfaces may present a risk of disease transmission under certain circumstances and these surfaces should be cleaned and disinfected consistently to minimize this risk. Although the major portion of the following discussion was written in 1978 pertaining only to sanitary practices that should be followed to prevent transmission of hepatitis type B, the current revision by the ad hoc Committee for Evaluation of Sanitary Practices in Cardiopulmonary Resuscitation Training is applicable to lessening the risks of transmitting a wide variety of infectious diseases.

There are several important infection control considerations in CPR training. First, the act of mouth-to-mouth or mouth-to-nose artificial respiration obviously requires close physical contact in which a potential rescuer must ignore his or her concerns for personal protection or aesthetic apprehensions to save the life of a victim. Accordingly, in training sessions, students are urged to overcome such hesitations, and they may practice on manikins contaminated by the hands and oral fluids of previous students. This situation becomes especially obvious during the practice of two-rescuer CPR in which the manikin cannot be adequately cleaned between uses by the the two students. Also, the practice of removing upper airway obstruction involves sweeping the back of the manikin throat with a finger, and in this situation, contamination from previous students may be smeared on the manikin face. In practice, there is usually no pause at this point to decontaminate the face before beginning mouth-to-mouth breathing (see recommendations that follow). Additionally, the valve mechanisms and lungs in manikin airways invariably become contaminated during use, and if they are not appropriately dismantled and cleaned after class, they may serve as contamination sources for subsequent classes. There is no recognized evidence, however, that the manikin valve mechanisms produce aerosols even when air is forcibly expelled during chest compression exercises.

Some manufacturers have provided protective face shields for manikins to improve hygienic conditions during training sessions, but it is unlikely that such shields would be changed after each use by students learning the two-rescuer resuscitation method. Protective shields and detailed instructions for sanitizing the manikins between uses by students and classes are available from several manufacturers.

When dealing with potential contamination by microorganisms having resistance levels that have not been fully characterized (e.g., AIDS, hepatitis and herpes viruses) the manikins pose a difficult disinfection problem. Although there are several intermediate- to high-level disinfectants recommended for use in instances of contamination such as hepatitis B,[68-70] the majority would meet with objection because of either material incompatibility with the manikin (e.g., staining or other damage of plastic materials by iodine compounds) or undesirable residues, odors, or toxicities that may affect students (e.g., formaldehyde, glutaraldehyde) when used during the training sessions. Alcohols, quaternary ammonium compounds, and phenolics are not generally recommended, since proper contact times for effective action are difficult to achieve (e.g., alcohols evaporate rapidly) or the compounds are not broad spectrum agents (e.g., quaternary ammonium compounds have limited action against certain viruses and bacteria).[70]

Recommendations

1. Purchasers of training manikins should thoroughly examine the manufacturers' recommendations and provisions for sanitary practices.

2. Students should be told in advance that the training sessions will involve "close physical contact" with their fellow students.

3. Students or instructors should not actively participate in training sessions (hands-on training with manikins) if they have dermatologic lesions on hands or in oral or circumoral areas, if they are known to be seropositive for hepatitis B surface antigen (HBsAg), if they have upper-respiratory-tract infections, if they have acquired immunodeficiency syndrome (AIDS), or if the student or instructor has reason to believe that he or she has been exposed to or is in the active stage of any infectious process.

4. If more than one CPR manikin is used in a particular training class, students should preferably be assigned in pairs, with each pair having contact with only one manikin. This would lessen the possible contamination of several manikins by one individual and therefore limit possible exposures of other class members.

5. All persons responsible for CPR training should be thoroughly familiar with hygienic concepts (e.g., thorough handwashing prior to manikin contact, not eating during class to avoid contamination of manikins with food particles, etc.), as well as the procedures for cleaning and maintaining manikins and accessories (e.g., face shields). Manikins should be inspected routinely for signs of physical deterioration, such as cracks or tears in plastic surfaces, which make thorough cleaning difficult or impossible. The clothes and hair of manikins should be washed periodically; e.g., monthly or whenever visibly soiled.

6. During the training of two-rescuer CPR, there is no opportunity to disinfect the manikin between students when the "switching procedure" is practiced. In order to limit the potential for disease transmission during this exercise, the second student taking over ventilation on the manikin should simulate ventilation

instead of blowing into the manikin. This recommendation is consistent with current training recommendations of the American Red Cross and the American Heart Association.

7. Training of the "obstructed airway procedure" involves the student using his or her finger to sweep foreign matter out of the manikin's mouth. This action could contaminate the student's finger with exhaled moisture and saliva from previous students in the same class and/or contaminate the manikin with material from the student's finger. When practicing this procedure, the finger sweep should either be simulated or done on a manikin whose airway was decontaminated before the procedure and will be decontaminated after the procedure.

8. At the end of each class, the procedures listed below should be followed as soon as possible to avoid drying of contamination on manikin surfaces. Personnel conducting the manikin disassembly and decontamination should wear protective latex gloves and wash their hands after finishing. (a) Disassemble manikin as directed by manufacturer. (b) As indicated, thoroughly wash all external and internal surfaces (also reusable protective face shields) with warm soapy water and brushes. (c) Rinse all surfaces with fresh water. (d) Wet all surfaces with a sodium hypochlorite solution having at least 500 ppm free available chlorine (1/4 cup liquid household bleach per gallon of tap water) for 10 minutes. This solution must be made fresh at each class and discarded after each use. (e) Rinse with fresh water and immediately dry all external and internal surfaces; rinsing with alcohol will aid drying of internal surfaces, and this drying will prevent the survival and growth of bacterial or fungal pathogens if the manikins are stored for periods longer than the day of cleaning.

9. Each time a different student uses the manikin in a training class, the individual protective face shield, if used, should be changed. Between students or after the instructor demonstrates a procedure such as clearing any obstruction from the airway, the manikin face and inside the mouth should be wiped vigorously with clean absorbent material (e.g., 4" by 4" gauze pad) wet with either the hypochlorite solution described in recommendation No. 8 (d) above or with 70% alcohol (isopropanol or ethanol). The surfaces should remain wet for at least 30 seconds before they are wiped dry with a second piece of clean absorbent material.

We are somewhat reluctant to recommend use of alcohols in this instance and do so only as an alternative, since some persons find the odor of hypochlorite objectionable. Although highly bactericidal, alcohols are not considered to be broad-spectrum agents and use of alcohols here is recommended primarily as an aid in mechanical cleaning; also, in a short contact period alcohols may not be effective against bacteria or other pathogens. Nonetheless, in the context of vigorous cleaning with alcohol and absorbent material, little viable microbial contamination of any kind is likely after the cleaning procedure.

10. People responsible for the use and maintenance of CPR manikins should be encouraged not to rely totally on the mere presence of a disinfectant to protect them and their students from cross-infection during training programs. Emphasis should be placed on the necessity of thorough physical cleaning (scrubbing, wiping) as the first step in an effective decontamination protocol. Microbial contamination is easily removed from smooth, nonporous surfaces by using disposable cleaning cloths moistened with a detergent solution, and there is no evidence that a soaking procedure alone in a liquid is as effective as the same procedure accompanied by vigorous scrubbing.

11. With specific regard to concerns about potential for hepatitis B and AIDS transmission in CPR training, it has recently been shown that the hepatitis B virus is not as resistant to disinfectant chemicals as it was once thought to be. Current recommendations for strategies dealing with AIDS contamination are the same as those for viral hepatitis B.[71-73]

In 1985 there was a dramatic increase in the number of inquiries regarding the adequacy of the current recommendation for manikin decontamination in killing the viral agent of the acquired immunodeficiency syndrome (AIDS). Recent studies have shown that the retroviral agent that causes AIDS, human T-cell lymphotrophic virus type III/lymphadenopathy-associated virus (HTLV-III/LAV), is comparatively delicate and is inactivated in less than ten minutes at room temperature by a number of disinfectant chemicals including the recommended agents, alcohol or sodium hypochlorite. Coupled with soap and water scrubbing and rinsing, the recommended sodium hypochlorite dilution will ensure that HTLV-III/LAV virus as well as a wide variety of other infectious agents with potential for contaminating manikin surfaces will be killed. In fact, if the steps in Recommendation 8 above are consistently followed, the students of each class should be presented with manikins having a sanitary quality equal to or better than eating utensils in a properly operated restaurant. A higher level of surface disinfection is not warranted and the recommended disinfectant chemicals (alcohol or household bleach) are safe, effective, inexpensive, easily obtained, and well tolerated by students, instructors, and manikin surfaces when properly used.

Current research and recommendations for HTLV-III/LAV contamination on surfaces has been published recently.[74-78] It is emphasized that there is no evidence to date that AIDS is transmitted either by casual personal contact, by indirect contact with inanimate surfaces, or by the airborne route.

The risk of transmission of any infectious disease by manikin practice appears to be low. While an estimated 40 million people in the United States and perhaps 150 million worldwide have been taught mouth-to-mouth breathing on manikins in the last 25 years, there has never been a documented case of transmission of bacterial, fungal, or viral disease by a CPR training manikin. Thus, in the absence of evidence of infectious disease risk, including risk for AIDS, the lifesaving potential of CPR should continue to be vigorously emphasized and energetic efforts in support of broad-scale CPR training should be continued.

Disease Transmission and Actual Performance of CPR

The vast majority of CPR performed in the United States is done by health care and public safety personnel, many of whom perform mouth-to-mouth ventilation frequently throughout the year on cardiac arrest victims about whom they have little or no medical information. An individual layperson is less likely to be in a situation to perform CPR than are health care personnel. A layperson who performs CPR is most likely to do so in the home (where 70% to 80% of cardiac arrests occur), commonly knows the cardiac arrest victim, and often has prior knowledge of the victim's health. There should be no reluctance by the rescuer in this situation to institute CPR.

The greatest concern over the theoretical risk of disease transmission from mouth-to-mouth resuscitation should be directed at individuals who perform CPR frequently, such as health care and public safety personnel, and prehospital emergency health care providers.

Providers of prehospital emergency health care include the following: paramedics, emergency medical technicians, law enforcement personnel, firefighters, lifeguards, and others whose jobs might require them to provide first-response medical care. The risk of transmission of infection ...from infected persons to providers of prehospital emergency health care should be no higher than that for HCWs [health care workers] providing emergency care in the hospital if appropriate precautions are taken to prevent exposure to blood or other body fluids. . . .

No transmission of HBV [hepatitis B virus] infection during mouth-to-mouth resuscitation has been documented. However, because of the theoretical risk of salivary transmission of HTLV-III/LAV during mouth-to-mouth resuscitation, special attention should be given to the use of disposable airway equipment or resuscitation bags and the wearing of gloves when in contact with blood or other body fluids. Resuscitation equipment and devices known or suspected to be contaminated with blood or other body fluids should be used once and disposed of or be thoroughly cleaned and disinfected after each use.[79]

Clear plastic face masks with one-way valves are available for use during mouth-to-mask ventilation. These masks provide diversion of the victim's exhaled gas away from the rescuer and may be used by health care providers and public safety personnel properly trained in their use during two-person rescue, in place of mouth-to-mouth ventilation. The need for and effectiveness of this adjunct in preventing transmission of an infectious disease during mouth-to-mouth ventilation are unknown. If this type of device is to be used as reassurance to the rescuer that a potential risk might be minimized, the rescuer must be adequately trained in its use, especially with respect to making an adequate seal on the face and maintaining a patent airway. Such a device would be applicable only to two-rescuer CPR, since it requires two hands to secure a proper face seal and to maintain an open airway. As an additional precaution the rescuer may elect to wear latex gloves since saliva or blood on the victim's mouth or face may be transferred to the rescuer's hands.

References

67. *Recommendations for Decontaminating Manikins Used in Cardiopulmonary Resuscitation: Hepatitis Surveillance,* report 42. Atlanta, Centers for Disease Control, 1978, pp 34–36.

68. Bond WW, Petersen NJ, Favero MS: Viral hepatitis B: Aspects of environmental control. *Health Lab Sci* 1977; 14:235–252.

69. Bond WW, Favero MS, Petersen NJ, et al: Inactivation of hepatitis B virus by intermediate- to high-level disinfectant chemicals. *J Clin Microbiol* 1983; 18:535–538.

70. Favero MS: Sterilization, disinfection and antisepsis in the hospital, in Lenette EH, Balows A, Hausler WJ Jr, et al (eds): *Manual of Clinical Microbiology*, ed 4. Washington, DC, American Society of Microbiology, 1985, pp 129–137.

71. Centers for Disease Control: Acquired immune deficiency syndrome (AIDS): Precautions for clinical and laboratory staffs. *MMWR* 1982; 31:577–580.

72. Centers for Disease Control: Prevention of acquired immune deficiency syndrome (AIDS): Report of inter-agency recommendations. *MMWR* 1983; 32:101–103.

73. Task Force on the Acquired Immunodeficiency Syndrome: Infection control guidelines for patients with acquired immunodeficiency syndrome (AIDS). *N. Engl J Med* 1983; 309:740 –744.

74. Bond WW: Inactivation of AIDS virus in clothing. *JAMA* 1985; 253:258.

75. Lettau LA, Bond WW, McDougal JS: Hepatitis and diaphragm fitting. *JAMA* 1985; 254:752.

76. Martin LS, McDougal JS, Loskoski SL: Disinfection and inactivation of the human T-lymphotrophic virus type III/ lymphadenopathy-associated virus. *J Infect Dis* 1985; 152:400 – 403.

77. McDougal JS, Cort SP, Kennedy MS, et al: Immunoassay for detection and quantitation of infectious viral particles of the human retrovirus lymphadenopathy-associated virus (LAV). *J Immunol Methods* 1985; 76:171–183.

78. Spire B, Dormont D, Barré-Sinoussi F, et al: Inactivation of lymphadenopathy-associated virus by heat, gamma rays and ultraviolet light. *Lancet* 1985; 1:188–189.

79. Recommendations for preventing transmission of infection with human T-lymphotrophic virus type III/lymphadenopathy-associated virus in the workplace. *MMWR* 1985; 34:681–696.

Journal of the American Medical Association, 262, no. 19 (November 17, 1989):2714–2715.

Risk of Infection During CPR Training and Rescue: Supplemental Guidelines

The American Heart Association and the American Red Cross used the findings from the 1985 National Conference on Standards and Guidelines for Cardiopulmonary Resuscitation and Emergency Cardiac Care to establish their policy on the risk of infection during cardiopulmonary resuscitation (CPR) training and rescue. Findings that support the safety of CPR training and rescue and appropriate risk reduction strategies are presented as an update to the 1985 article. The Emergency Cardiac Care Committee of the American Heart Association incorporated recent advisories from the Centers for Disease Control as well as other information into guidelines that augment earlier recommendations.

(*JAMA.* 1989;262:2714–2715)

FINDINGS from the 1985 National Conference on Standards and Guidelines for Cardiopulmonary Resuscitation and Emergency Cardiac Care are the basis of the official position of both the American Heart Association and the American Red Cross on risk of infections during cardiopulmonary resuscitation (CPR) training and rescue. These guidelines[1] have been augmented by advisories from the Centers for Disease Control released in 1987[2] and 1988[3] and from the National Institute of Occupational Safety and Health in 1989.[4]

The Emergency Cardiac Care Committee of the American Heart Association considered specific issues related to risk of infection associated with both training and on-site rescue. The American Heart Association and the American Red Cross recommend the following guidelines for adoption.

GUIDELINES FOR RESCUERS WITH KNOWN OR SUSPECTED INFECTIONS

Transmission of hepatitis B virus (HBV) between health care workers and patients has been documented. Instruments and patients' open wounds have been contaminated when health care workers with high concentrations of HBV (much higher than that achieved in human immunodeficiency virus [HIV] infections) in their blood sustained a puncture wound while performing invasive procedures or had weeping lesions or small lacerations on their hands. Transmission of HIV from patients to health care workers has been documented in cases of blood exchange or penetration of the skin by blood-contaminated instruments.[5]

Direct mouth-to-mouth resuscitation will likely result in exchange of saliva between victim and rescuer. Hepatitis B-positive saliva has not been shown to be infectious, however, when applied to oral mucous membranes or through contamination of shared musical instruments or CPR training mannequins used by hepatitis B carriers. In addition, saliva has not been implicated in the transmission of HIV after bites, percutaneous inoculation, or contamination of cuts and open wounds with saliva from HIV-infected patients.[6,7]

Performance of mouth-to-mouth resuscitation or invasive procedures can result in exchange of blood between victim and rescuer if either has had breaks in the skin on or around the lips or soft tissues of the oral cavity mucosa. Thus, there is a theoretical risk of HBV and HIV transmission during mouth-to-mouth resuscitation.[8] It is important to note that the theoretical risk of infection is greater for salivary or aerosol transmission of herpes simplex and *Neisseria meningitidis* and for transmission of airborne diseases such as tuberculosis and respiratory infections.

- *Regardless of the type of infection, rescuers who have an infection that may be transmitted by blood or saliva or who believe they have been exposed to such an infection should not perform mouth-to-mouth resuscitation if circumstances allow other immediate or effective methods of ventilation, such as use of a bag-valve mask.*

GUIDELINES FOR RESCUERS WITH A DUTY TO PROVIDE CPR

The probability of a rescuer's becoming infected with HBV or HIV as a result of performing CPR is minimal.[4] To date, transmission of HBV or HIV infection during mouth-to-mouth resuscitation has not been documented.[9] However, to minimize the risk of transmitting a variety of diseases, mechanical ventilation or barrier devices should be accessible to those asked to provide CPR in the course of their employment. This includes emergency medical service personnel, firefighters, police, and lifeguards, as well as hospital and clinic health care workers.

Although efficacy in preventing disease transmission has not been demonstrated conclusively, masks with one-way valves and bag-valve devices are available, and those with a duty to respond should be instructed in their use during training. Plastic mouth and nose covers with filtered openings also are available and *may* provide a degree of protection against transfer of oral fluids and aerosols. Masks without one-way valves (including those with S-shaped mouthpieces) and handkerchiefs offer little, if any, protection and should not be considered for routine use. Intubation obviates the need for mouth-to-mouth resuscitation and is more effective than the use of bag-mask devices. Early intubation should be encouraged when equipment and trained professionals are available.

• *Individuals with a duty to respond are reminded of their moral, ethical, and, in certain situations, legal obligations to provide CPR, especially in the occupational setting.*

GUIDELINES FOR THE LAYPERSON

The layperson who responds in an emergency should be guided by individual moral and ethical values and knowledge of risks that may exist in various rescue situations. It is safest for the rescuer to assume that all emergency situations that involve transfer of certain body fluids have the potential for disease transmission for both rescuer and victim.

Intact skin is the primary defense against transmission of blood-borne diseases during CPR. Transmission of HBV or HIV is more likely if the rescuer has lesions, cuts, or sores in or around the mouth or on the hands and has contact with the victim's blood, vomitus that contains blood, and/or saliva that contains blood. A rescuer who believes he or she has had parenteral or mucous membrane contact with the victim's blood or blood-contaminated body fluids should wash promptly and thoroughly and contact a physician.

• *As a minimum action, in situations perceived as high-risk for disease transmission, the lay rescuer should assess the victim's responsiveness, call for help, position the victim, open the airway, and, in the absence of a pulse, perform chest compressions.*[10] *However, the rescuer should remember that delayed ventilation could mean death or disablement for an otherwise healthy person, while risk to the rescuer, even with a known HBV/HIV-positive victim, is considered very low.*

CPR TRAINING FOR INFECTED INDIVIDUALS

To date, transmission of HBV infection through use of CPR mannequins by HBV carriers has not been shown. Neither has saliva been implicated in HIV transmission. Because of potential breakdown of oral and circumoral mucosa during practice on a mannequin, however, CPR training poses a theoretical risk to class participants. It is recommended that students and instructors adhere to the guidelines that follow.

Acute Infections or Dermatologic Lesions

Acute respiratory infections such as the common cold run a short course, and most breaks in the skin heal naturally or after medical attention. Therefore, students or instructors should postpone CPR training if they (1) are known to be in the active stage of an infection, (2) have reason to believe they have been exposed to an infectious disease, or (3) have dermatologic lesions on their hands or in oral or circumoral areas.

Chronic Infections

Chronic infections such as HBV and HIV persist over an extended period and can be transmitted even when the carrier is asymptomatic. If an instructor wishes to train or to present course completion cards to an individual with a known chronic infection or if the instructor has a known chronic infection, precautions must be taken to protect other participants from exposure. This is best accomplished by providing the infected individual with a separate mannequin that is not used by anyone else until it has been cleaned according to recommended end-of-class decontamination procedures.

- *An individual who has an acute or chronic infection that may be transmitted by blood or saliva must not participate in CPR training until his or her personal physician has reviewed the circumstances carefully and indicated whether participation is appropriate. Because CPR course participants may not know that they have been exposed to an infection, it is imperative that participants and instructors adhere strictly to established procedures for decontamination of the mannequin.*[11] *In addition, requests for individual mannequins should be honored, within reason. Equitable accommodations for all participants in CPR programs are encouraged.*

EDUCATION FOR THE CHRONICALLY INFECTED RESCUER

Individuals with chronic infections should be educated about potential transmission of infection to victims during CPR. Course participants should be made aware of guidelines for rescuers with known or suspected infections. Health risks to the chronically infected rescuer also should be emphasized. If the rescuer's immune system has been altered by any cause, performance of CPR may pose a greater risk to the rescuer. Contact with a victim who is in the active stage of an infection (eg, influenza, tuberculosis, HBV infection, and other respiratory infections) may jeopardize the health of the rescuer with depressed immune function.

GUIDELINES FOR INDIVIDUALS UNABLE TO COMPLETE A CPR COURSE

It is the position of the American Heart Association and the American Red Cross that all reasonable accommodations should be made to provide CPR training to anyone who desires it. It is understood, however, that not everyone will be able to meet the standards required for completion of a CPR course. Such individuals include, but are not limited to, those with physical disabilities that prevent acute ventilation of a mannequin or patient, those unable to perform adequate chest compressions, and those with chronic infections. This may create a dilemma for an individual whose job requires CPR course completion.

Whether an infected worker can care for patients adequately and safely must be determined on an individual basis. The worker's personal physician should make this decision in conjunction with the employing agency and its medical advisers.

- *It is not the role of the American Heart Association or the American Red Cross to lower their course completion standards to accommodate, for purposes of employment, individuals unable to meet these standards. This is an issue that must be resolved by the employer and the employee; thus, the employer must decide whether to waive the CPR course completion requirement. The more important issue for someone who is unable to complete the desired course is whether he or she is able to work in a situation that requires administration of CPR.*

Approved by the Steering Committee of the American Heart Association.

References

1. Standards and guidelines for cardiopulmonary resuscitation and emergency cardiac care. *JAMA*. 1986;255:2905–3044.
2. Centers for Disease Control. Recommendations for prevention of HIV transmission in health-care settings. *MMWR*. 1987;36 (suppl 2):1S–18S.
3. Centers for Disease Control. Update: universal precautions for prevention of transmission of human immunodeficiency virus, hepatitis B virus, and other bloodborne pathogens in health-care settings. *MMWR*. 1988;37:377–382, 387–388.
4. Centers for Disease Control. Guidelines for prevention of transmission of human immunodeficiency virus and hepatitis

B virus to health-care and public safety workers. *MMWR.* 1989;38(suppl 6):1–37.
5. Marcus R, the CDC Cooperative Needlestick Surveillance Group. Surveillance of health care workers exposed to blood from patients infected with human immunodeficiency virus. *N Engl J Med.* 1988;319:1118–1123.
6. Fox PC, Wolff A, Yeh CK, Atkinson JC, Baum BJ. Saliva inhibits HIV-1 infectivity. *J Am Dent Assoc.* 1988;116:635–637.
7. Friedland GH, Saltzman BR, Rogers MF, Lesser ML, Mayers MM, Klein RS. Lack of transmission of HTLV III/LAV infection to household contacts of patients with AIDS or AIDS-related complex with oral candidiasis. *N Engl J Med.* 1986;314:344–349.
8. Piazza M, Chirianni A, Picciotto L, Guadagnino V, Orlando R, Cataldo PT. Passionate kissing and microlesions of the oral mucosa: possible role in AIDS transmission. *JAMA.* 1989;261:244–245.
9. Sande MA. Transmission of AIDS: the case against causal contagion. *N Engl J Med.* 1986;314:380–382.
10. Lesser R, Bircher N, Safar P, Stezoski W. Sternal compression before ventilation in cardiopulmonary resuscitation (CPR). *J World Assoc Emerg Disaster Med.* 1985;1(suppl 1):239–241.
11. Centers for Disease Control. *Understanding AIDS: A Message From the Surgeon General.* Washington, DC: US Dept of Health and Human Services; 1988.

Appendix B

Written Exams, Answer Sheet, Answer Keys, and Scoring Keys

This appendix contains—

- Two 70-item exams—Exam A and Exam B
- A blank 70-item answer sheet
- Two answer keys—one for each exam

Note: Two scoring keys, one for each exam, are at the end of this manual, after the index.

Exam Specifications

Textbook Chapter		Number of Questions
Chapter 1	The Citizen Responder	3
Chapter 2	Body Systems	4
Chapter 3	Responding to Emergencies	9
Chapter 4	Breathing Emergencies	7
Chapter 5	Cardiac Emergencies	7
Chapter 6	Bleeding	2
Chapter 7	Shock	3
Chapter 8	Soft Tissue Injuries	4
Chapter 9	Musculoskeletal Injuries	4
Chapter 10	Injuries to the Head and Spine	3
Chapter 11	Injuries to the Chest, Abdomen, and Pelvis	3
Chapter 12	Injuries to the Extremities	2
Chapter 13	Sudden Illnesses	4
Chapter 14	Poisoning, Bites, and Stings	3
Chapter 15	Substance Misuse and Abuse	3
Chapter 16	Heat and Cold Exposure	4
Chapter 17	Reaching and Moving Victims	2
Chapter 18	Your Guide to a Healthier Life	3
	TOTAL	**70 QUESTIONS**

Either exam A or exam B may be used. However, if a participant fails the initial exam, then use the other exam for a retest. For example, if a participant fails exam A, she or she should review the textbook and then be retested using exam B.

Some participants may have difficulty with any written exam even though they understand the course material. In such cases, you may administer the test orally by reading the questions aloud. Oral exams should not be given until all other participants have completed the written exam. (See Chapter 5 in this manual.)

American Red Cross First Aid—Responding to Emergencies Exam A

IMPORTANT: Read all instructions before beginning this exam.

INSTRUCTIONS: Mark all answers in pencil on a separate answer sheet. Do not write on this exam. The questions on this exam are multiple choice. Read each question slowly and carefully. Then choose the **best** answer and fill in that circle on the answer sheet. If you wish to change an answer, erase your first answer completely. Return this exam to your instructor when you are finished.

EXAMPLE

ANSWER SHEET

75. 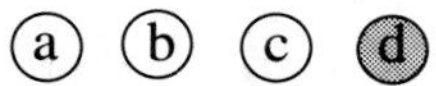  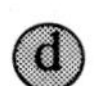

75. Why does the American Red Cross teach this first aid course?
    a. To help people stay calm in emergencies
    b. To help people make appropriate decisions when they confront and emergency
    c. To help people in an emergency keep a victim's injuries from getting worse until EMS arrives
    d. All of the above

1. Which of the following statements best describe the emergency medical services (EMS) system?
   a. The EMS system provides an ambulance to transport the victim to the hospital.
   b. The EMS system consists of community resources organized to care for victims of sudden illness or injury.
   c. Personnel and equipment for removing victims from dangerous locations are part of the EMS system.
   d. The EMS system is organized to prevent the occurrence of injuries and sudden illness.

2. As a citizen responder, which is your most important responsibility in a life-threatening situation?
   a. Summoning EMS professionals
   b. Getting others to help you
   c. Moving the victim to safety
   d. Taking the victim to the hospital

3. Which of the following is a barrier to action in an emergency?
   a. Not wanting to get involved for fear of doing something wrong.
   b. Uncertainty about providing first aid due to the nature of the injury or illness.
   c. Embarrassment about stepping forward to provide first aid in front of strangers.
   d. All of the above

4. The heart, blood, and blood vessels are major components of which body system?
   a. Nervous
   b. Integumentary
   c. Circulatory
   d. Musculoskeletal

5. In reaction to cold, the skin becomes pale and shows what is called "gooseflesh." Which two systems are interacting with the skin to maintain body temperature?
   a. Nervous, musculoskeletal
   b. Respiratory, integumentary
   c. Circulatory, musculoskeletal
   d. Nervous, circulatory

6. Which two body systems function with the alveoli to provide oxygen for the cells of the body?
   a. Musculoskeletal, integumentary
   b. Respiratory, circulatory
   c. Integumentary, respiratory
   d. Circulatory, musculoskeletal

7. The pain that accompanies a burn from hot water is an example of the interrelationship of which body systems?
   a. Respiratory, musculoskeletal
   b. Circulatory, respiratory
   c. Musculoskeletal, integumentary
   d. Integumentary, nervous

8. Which step of the emergency action principles should you take first?
   a. Doing a primary survey.
   b. Doing a secondary survey.
   c. Surveying the scene.
   d. Calling EMS personnel for help.

9. Why should you follow the emergency action principles?
   a. They ensure that necessary care is provided in any emergency.
   b. They provide you with a detailed medical history for the victim.
   c. They lead you to a diagnosis of the victim's illness or injury.
   d. None of the above

10. A car has crashed into a power pole and a live electrical wire is draped over its roof. The driver of the car is slumped against the steering wheel and appears to be bleeding heavily from a facial injury. What should be your immediate action in this situation?
    a. Approach the driver and determine if he is conscious and breathing.
    b. Move the live wire off the car using rubber gloves and a dry branch or pole.
    c. Stay back from the car and call EMS personnel to deal with the situation.
    d. Instruct the driver to carefully open the door and jump clear of the car.

11. To which of these victims can you provide first aid because consent is implied?
    a. An unconscious victim
    b. An unaccompanied infant or child
    c. A victim unable to respond due to illness or injury.
    d. All of the above

12. Why should you do a primary survey in every emergency situation?
    a. Because it protects you from legal liability
    b. Because it identifies conditions that are an immediate threat to life
    c. Because it identifies conditions that could become life-threatening if not cared for
    d. Because it enables you to protect the victim and bystanders from dangers at the scene

13. In what order do you assess the four elements of a primary survey? (first to last)
    a. Airway, breathing, circulation, consciousness
    b. Breathing, airway, circulation, consciousness
    c. Circulation, consciousness, airway, breathing
    d. Consciousness, airway, breathing, circulation

14. For which of the following people should you **immediately** summon EMS personnel?
    a. A 22-year-old male who has had a fever and vomited twice during the night.
    b. A 60-year-old jogger experiencing severe knee pain after a morning run
    c. A 40-year-old executive complaining that he has felt nauseated, sweaty, and weak for the past hour or so
    d. An 8-year-old with a large bruise on one arm from being hit by a baseball

15. To which of the following should you give special attention during a secondary survey?
    a. Identification cards found in the victim's wallet
    b. A medical-alert bracelet
    c. The name and address of the victim's next of kin
    d. Cash and credit cards carried by the victim

16. Which victim might it be appropriate for you to transport to the hospital?
    a. A 42-year-old man complaining of chest pain that comes and goes.
    b. A 10-year-old girl who fell from her bicycle and has an open fracture of the forearm.
    c. A 50-year-old man whose hand was slammed in a door and is swollen, and painful.
    d. None of the above

17. When you give rescue breathing, you are—
    a. Supplying the victim with oxygen necessary for survival.
    b. Supplementing the air the victim is already breathing.
    c. Artificially circulating oxygen-rich blood to the body cells.
    d. All of the above

18. Which must you do to determine if a victim requires rescue breathing?
    a. Check for a pulse in the neck.
    b. Look, listen, and feel for breathing.
    c. Check for bluish or grayish skin color.
    d. All of the above

19. Which is the most dependable method of evaluating the effectiveness of rescue breathing?
    a. Assuring that your mouth is sealed securely against the victim's mouth
    b. Assuring that the victim's nose is pinched securely shut
    c. Breathing into the victim's mouth for exactly 1 to 1 1/2 seconds
    d. Seeing the victim's chest rise with each breath you deliver

20. How can you minimize the amount of air forced into a victim's stomach during rescue breathing?
    a. Breathe slowly into the victim when delivering breaths.
    b. Do not pause between breaths unless absolutely necessary.
    c. Press on the victim's stomach while delivering breaths.
    d. Breathe as hard as you can into the victim.

21. After discovering that your first two breaths are not causing the victim's chest to rise, what should you do?
    a. Call EMS personnel.
    b. Do a finger sweep.
    c. Give two more breaths with more force.
    d. Retilt the head and give breaths again.

22. After giving your first series of 6 to 10 abdominal thrusts to an unconscious victim with an obstructed airway, you should—
    a. Do a finger sweep and then give 2 full breaths.
    b. Give 2 full breaths and then do a finger sweep.
    c. Check for pulse, give 2 full breaths, and do a finger sweep.
    d. Do a finger sweep and check for pulse.

23. While eating dinner, a friend suddenly starts to cough weakly and make high-pitched noises. You should—
    a. Lower him to the floor, do a finger sweep, give 2 full breaths and 6 to 10 abdominal thrusts.
    b. Give abdominal thrusts until the object is dislodged or he becomes unconscious.
    c. Encourage him to continue coughing to try to dislodge the object.
    d. Open the airway using the head-tilt/chin-lift.

24. Which is the key signal of a heart attack?
    a. Difficulty breathing
    b. Pain in the jaw and left arm
    c. Nausea and sweating
    d. Persistent chest pain

25. Which is your most important responsibility in caring for a victim complaining of shortness of breath and pressure in the chest?
    a. Having the victim stop what he is doing and rest in a comfortable position
    b. Providing CPR
    c. Recognizing that these signals may indicate a heart attack
    d. Asking the victim about previous medical conditions and helping him take nitroglycerine if prescribed

26. Which is the primary signal of cardiac arrest?
    a. Absence of a radial pulse
    b. No breathing
    c. Dilation of the pupils
    d. Absence of a carotid pulse

27. Which is the purpose of cardiopulmonary resuscitation (CPR)?
    a. To restart heartbeat and breathing in a victim of cardiac arrest
    b. To keep the brain supplied with oxygen until the heart can be restarted
    c. To prevent clinical death from occurring in a victim of cardiac arrest
    d. All of the above

28. When should you stop providing CPR?
    I. When EMS personnel take over
    II. When a neighbor tells you to stop
    III. When you are exhausted
    IV. If the scene becomes unsafe
    V. If the victim vomits

    ---

    a. I, III, and IV
    b. II and IV
    c. V only
    d. All of the above

29. High blood pressure can be controlled by—
    a. Losing excess weight.
    b. Taking prescribed medication.
    c. Changing dietary habits.
    d. All of the above

30. Which of the following is a risk factor for heart disease that cannot be controlled?
    a. High blood pressure
    b. Heredity
    c. Smoking
    d. Cholesterol level

31. How can you minimize the risk of disease transmission when controlling external bleeding?
    a. Wash your hands before and immediately after giving care.
    b. Minimize direct contact with blood.
    c. Use protective barriers such as gloves or plastic wrap.
    d. All of the above

32. What should you do for a victim who appears to have serious internal bleeding?
    a. Call EMS personnel.
    b. Place the victim in a sitting position.
    c. Give fluids to drink to replace blood loss.
    d. Apply heat to the injured area.

33. Which signal is often the first indicator that the body is experiencing a problem that may result in shock?
    a. Nausea and vomiting
    b. Loss of consciousness
    c. Restlessness or irritability
    d. Pale or bluish, cool, moist skin

34. Why does the skin of a victim in shock appear pale and feel cool?
    a. Because shock damages the temperature control centers in the brain and spinal cord
    b. Because the body responds to shock by reducing the amount of blood going to the skin
    c. Because shock causes the heart to slow, reducing the amount of heat generated by the body
    d. Because the body responds to shock by cooling itself to decrease energy needs

35. Which is the appropriate position for a victim who is showing the signals of shock as a result of injuries to the head and neck?
    a. Legs elevated about 24 inches
    b. Head and shoulders elevated about 12 inches
    c. Lying flat on the back
    d. On one side with head slightly elevated

36. Which of the following signals indicate that a wound in the palm of the hand is infected?
    I. Tingling in the fingertips
    II. Redness and warmth in the palm
    III. Stiffness in the elbow
    IV. Throbbing pain in the palm and wrist
    V. Red streaks on the inner forearm
    VI. Bluish tinge to the nail beds

    ---

    a. All of the above
    b. III, IV, and V
    c. II, IV, and V
    d. I, II, and VI

37. Which of the following guidelines should you follow when applying a bandage?
    I. Leave a corner of the dressing exposed to check it for blood saturation.
    II. Elevate the injured part above the level of the heart, if safe to do so.
    III. Do not cover the fingers or toes unless absolutely necessary.
    IV. Remove and replace a dressing which becomes saturated with blood.
    V. Loosen the bandage slightly if fingers or toes below the bandage become pale.

    ---

    a. All of the above
    b. I and IV
    c. II, III, IV, and V
    d. II, III, and V

38. Caring for an infected wound includes—
    a. Keeping the area uncovered.
    b. Seeking medical help if the infection persists.
    c. Applying cool, wet compresses.
    d. All of the above

39. Burns that require professional medical attention—
    a. Are only those that affect the limbs.
    b. Are those resulting from electricity, explosions, or chemicals.
    c. Are burns whose victims are having difficulty breathing.
    d. b and c

40. In which of the following musculoskeletal injuries is there usually no apparent deformity?
    a. Fracture
    b. Dislocation
    c. Strain
    d. All of the above

41. You should suspect a serious musculoskeletal injury if the victim tells you that she—
    a. Has a slight pain in her ankle when she walks.
    b. Heard a snap or pop when she struck the ground.
    c. Has a history of frequent prior dislocations.
    d. Notices that her injured wrist feels warm to the touch.

42. Which of the following are included in your general care for musculoskeletal injuries?
    a. Rest, ice, and elevation
    b. Ice and gentle exercise
    c. Splints, bandaging, and elevation
    d. Rest and heat packs

43. An effective splint should do all of the following **except-**
    a. Prevent a closed fracture from becoming an open fracture.
    b. Decrease circulation to the injured area and minimize swelling.
    c. Lessen pain and increase the victim's comfort.
    d. Reduce the risk of serious internal bleeding.

44. For which of the following people should you consider the possibility of a serious head and/or spinal injury?
    a. An 18-year-old who fell from a height of 3 feet
    b. A helmeted motorcyclist whose helmet was cracked as he hit the ground
    c. A conscious victim of a motor vehicle crash who was not wearing a seat belt
    d. b and c

45. Which is often the first and most important signal of a serious head injury?
    a. Blood or fluid in the ears
    b. Altered level of consciousness
    c. Severe pain or pressure in the head
    d. Seizures or convulsions

46. From which part of the body should you remove an impaled object if necessary to control bleeding?
    a. Cheek
    b. Chest
    c. Eye
    d. Hand

47. Which should be included in your basic care for serious chest or abdominal injuries?
    I. Calling EMS personnel
    II. Administering oxygen
    III. Applying ice or cold packs
    IV. Minimizing shock
    V. Limiting victim movement

    ---

    a. I, II, and IV
    b. II and V
    c. I, III, IV, and V
    d. I, IV, and V

48. Which signals indicate possible serious abdominal injury?
    I. Nausea and vomiting
    II. Respiratory distress
    III. Weakness and thirst
    IV. Coughing blood
    V. Bruising

    ---

    a. I and II
    b. III and IV
    c. I, III, and V
    d. II and III

49. Which of the following is part of the first aid care for a victim of a suspected pelvic fracture?
    a. Rolling the victim to a position lying flat on the back
    b. Placing the victim on one side with the knees flexed toward the abdomen
    c. Moving the victim to a semisitting position unless pain is increased
    d. Not moving the victim from the position found unless necessary

50. A child has fallen from a skateboard and landed on an elbow. What signals would you expect to see if the elbow is seriously injured?
    I. Pain in the wrist
    II. Deformity at the elbow
    III. Swelling and discoloration of the elbow
    IV. Paralysis of the hand

    ---

    a. All of the above
    b. I and IV
    c. II and III
    d. I, II, and III

51. How should you immobilize a serious shoulder injury?
    a. Allow the victim to continue to support the arm and immobilize it in that position.
    b. Gently straighten the arm, apply a rigid splint, and secure it to the victim's body.
    c. Use pillows, blankets, or other padding to fill any gaps between the arm and the victim's body.
    d. a and c

52. Your first aid care for a victim of fainting should include—
    I. Placing the victim in a semisitting position.
    II. Elevating the victim's legs.
    III. Giving a conscious victim small sips of water or fruit juice.
    IV. Conducting a primary survey.
    V. Splashing water on the victim's face.

    ---

    a. I, III, and V
    b. II and IV
    c. I and III
    d. II, IV, and V

53. Which of the following are considered general signals of sudden illness?
    a. Change in level of consciousness
    b. Slowing pulse and breathing rates
    c. Nausea and vomiting
    d. All of the above

54. A friend who is a diabetic is drowsy and seems confused. He is not sure if he took his insulin that day. What should you do?
    a. Give him some sugar.
    b. Suggest he rest for an hour or so.
    c. Tell him to take his insulin.
    d. b and c

55. In caring for a victim having a seizure, you should—
    a. Try to hold the person still.
    b. Move any objects that might cause injury.
    c. Place a spoon between the person's teeth.
    d. Douse the person with water.

56. In which of the following ingested poisoning situations might the Poison Control Center tell you to induce a victim to vomit?
    a. Less than 30 minutes has passed since the poisoning.
    b. More than 3 hours has passed since the poisoning.
    c. The poison is a petroleum product.
    d. The victim is unconscious.

57. How should you remove a stinger embedded in a victim's skin?
    a. Use a tweezers to pull it out.
    b. Scrape it away from the skin with a fingernail or plastic card.
    c. Use a small sewing needle to pull it from the skin.
    d. Any of the above techniques is acceptable.

58. Which will help protect you from insect and tick bites?
    - I. Wearing long-sleeved shirts and long pants in wooded areas
    - II. Walking or hiking early in the morning or around dusk
    - III. Taping the area where your pants and socks meet
    - IV. Wearing dark clothes, which are less attractive to insects and ticks
    - V. Spraying repellent on pets that go outdoors

    ---

    a. All of the above
    b. II, IV, and V
    c. I, III, and V
    d. I, II, and III

59. To avoid an unintentional misuse or overdose of a prescription drug, you should know the—
    a. Effects of the drug.
    b. Potential side effects of the drug.
    c. Drugs with which it will interact.
    d. All of the above

60. Which of the following is true of substance abuse?
    a. It occurs only among the elderly who are forgetful and may have poor eyesight.
    b. It is the use of a substance for intended purposes but in improper amounts or doses.
    c. It is the use of a substance without regard to health concerns or accepted medical practices.
    d. Its effects are minor and rarely result in medical complications.

61. You are walking home from a movie and notice a man in front of you stumble and fall. He gets to his feet and walks unsteadily toward you. You ask him if he is alright and he replies incoherently. He stumbles again and falls. Which of the conditions below could cause this person's problems?
    a. Depressant overdose
    b. Alcohol intoxication
    c. Hyperglycemia
    d. All of the above

62. Which first aid care should you provide for a victim of hypothermia?
    I. Remove any wet clothing and dry the victim.
    II. Immerse the victim in warm water, if possible.
    III. Give warm liquids to drink, if the victim is conscious.
    IV. Closely monitor the victim's condition.
    V. Handle the victim gently.

    a. I, II, and V
    b. II, III, and IV
    c. I, III, IV, and V
    d. All of the above

63. As you are providing first aid to a victim of heat-related illness, which signals indicate that you should immediately call EMS personnel?
    a. The victim refuses water or vomits.
    b. The victim loses consciousness.
    c. The victim begins to sweat profusely.
    d. a and b

64. If the victim of a suspected heat-related illness begins to lose consciousness, you should—
    a. Cool the body using wet sheets, towels, or cold packs.
    b. Cool the body by applying rubbing alcohol.
    c. Give cool water to drink.
    d. a and c

65. Precautions you can take that will help you prevent both heat- and cold-related illnesses include—
    a. Keeping a constant, measured pace of activity while outdoors.
    b. Always wearing appropriate clothing for the environment.
    c. Drinking plenty of fluids.
    d. b and c

66. In which of the following situations would you move a victim before providing first aid care?
    a. A victim lying in a supermarket aisle where a large crowd has gathered obstructing the aisle.
    b. A victim unconscious in his car in a closed garage; the car's engine is running.
    c. A victim who has fallen on her back in the bleachers at a high school football game; it is raining.
    d. A victim sitting in his truck on the shoulder of a busy highway; the truck's engine is running.

67. How can you help protect a victim from further injury when moving him or her in an emergency?
    a. Move the victim in a sitting position whenever possible
    b. Roll the victim rather than pulling him from the head or feet
    c. Keep the victim's head and neck supported during the movement
    d. All of the above

68. A 25-year-old woman is starting a cardiovascular fitness program. What Target Heart Rate (THR) should she seek to achieve during exercise?
    a. 108 to 126 beats per minute
    b. 127 to 156 beats per minute
    c. 146 to 175 beats per minute
    d. 165 to 195 beats per minute

69. Smoking increases the risk of—
    I. Lung cancer.
    II. Diabetes.
    III. Heart attack.
    IV. Stomach ulcers.

    ---

    a. I and III
    b. II and IV
    c. I, II, and III
    d. All of the above

70. To avoid reaching a level of blood alcohol that impairs judgement and reflexes, you should limit yourself to—
    a. Three drinks per hour.
    b. Two drinks per hour.
    c. One drink per hour.
    d. Four drinks per hour.

American Red Cross First Aid—Responding to Emergencies Exam B

IMPORTANT: Read all instructions before beginning this exam.

INSTRUCTIONS: Mark all answers in pencil on a separate answer sheet. Do not write on this exam. The questions on this exam are multiple choice. Read each question slowly and carefully. Then choose the **best** answer and fill in that circle on the answer sheet. If you wish to change an answer, erase your first answer completely. Return this exam to your instructor when you are finished.

EXAMPLE

ANSWER SHEET

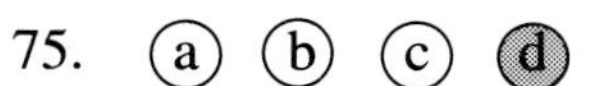

75. Why does the American Red Cross teach this first aid course?

    a. To help people stay calm in emergencies

    b. To help people make appropriate decisions when they confront and emergency

    c. To help people in an emergency keep a victim's injuries from getting worse until EMS arrives

    d. All of the above

1. Which of the following statements best describe the emergency medical services (EMS) system?
   a. The EMS system consists of community resources organized to care for victims of sudden illness or injury.
   b. The EMS system provides an ambulance to transport the victim to the hospital.
   c. Personnel and equipment for removing victims from dangerous locations are part of the EMS system.
   d. The EMS system is organized to prevent the occurrence of injuries and sudden illness.

2. As a citizen responder, which is your most important responsibility in a life-threatening situation?
   a. Getting others to help you
   b. Moving the victim to safety
   c. Summoning EMS professionals
   d. Taking the victim to the hospital

3. If a victim's behavior threatens your safety while you are attempting to provide first aid, what should you do?
   a. Try to restrain the victim and prevent harm to yourself and others.
   b. Attempt to calm the victim by gently touching his or her arm and talking softly.
   c. Try speaking forcefully and authoritatively to the victim to gain cooperation.
   d. Withdraw from the immediate area and wait for EMS professionals.

4. The heart, blood, and blood vessels are major components of which body system?
   a. Circulatory
   b. Integumentary
   c. Musculoskeletal
   d. Nervous

5. Which structure listed below is part of the integumentary system?
   a. Muscle
   b. Skin
   c. Bone
   d. Nerves

6. The respiratory system works with other body systems to provide oxygen to all body cells. These systems include the—
   a. Circulatory and nervous systems.
   b. Nervous system.
   c. Musculoskeletal, nervous, and circulatory systems.
   d. Musculoskeletal and circulatory systems.

7. The human body rapidly adapts to new environments. For example, when you step outside of an air-conditioned building on a hot, summer day, you immediately begin to sweat. Your body adapts to its "new" environment. What systems work together to produce this specific adaptation?
   a. Nervous and musculoskeletal systems
   b. Integumentary and respiratory systems
   c. Circulatory and respiratory systems
   d. Integumentary and nervous systems

8. Why should you follow the emergency action principles?
   a. They lead you to a diagnosis of the victim's illness or injury.
   b. They provide you with a detailed medical history for the victim.
   c. They ensure that necessary care is provided in any emergency.
   d. None of the above

9. A car has crashed into a power pole and a live electrical wire is draped over its roof. The driver of the car is slumped against the steering wheel and appears to be bleeding heavily from a facial injury. What should be your immediate action in this situation?
   a. Stay back from the car and call EMS personnel to deal with the situation.
   b. Move the live wire off the car using rubber gloves and a dry branch or pole.
   c. Instruct the driver to carefully open the door and jump clear of the car.
   d. Approach the driver and determine if he is conscious and breathing.

10. To which of these victims can you provide first aid because consent is implied.
    a. An unaccompanied infant or child
    b. An unconscious victim
    c. A victim unable to respond due to illness or injury
    d. All of the above

11. In addition to identifying yourself and your level of training to a conscious victim, what else must you tell the victim in order to obtain his or her consent to first aid care?
    a. Which ambulance service you are calling
    b. Where you received your training
    c. What you would like to do
    d. What you think is wrong with the victim

12. For which of the following people should you **immediately** summon EMS personnel?
    a. A 40-year-old executive complaining that he has felt nauseated, sweaty, and weak for the past hour or so
    b. A 60-year-old jogger experiencing severe knee pain after a morning run
    c. A 22-year-old male who has had a fever and vomited twice during the night
    d. An 8-year-old with a large bruise on one arm from being hit by a baseball

13. Which of the following conditions would you discover in a secondary survey?
    a. Cardiac arrest
    b. Open fracture with severe bleeding
    c. Allergies to bee stings and penicillin
    d. All of the above

14. If you decide to transport a victim to the hospital yourself, what precautions should you take?
    a. Have a bystander call the hospital and report the victim's condition.
    b. Make certain that the victim is transported lying down.
    c. Have a bystander notify the police to ask an officer to meet you at the hospital.
    d. Take a second person with you to ensure that the victim is constantly observed.

15. Why is it necessary to complete a primary survey in every emergency situation?
    a. To check for minor injuries
    b. To determine if there are any life-threatening conditions that need immediate care
    c. To get consent from the victim before providing care
    d. To ask for information about the cause of the illness or injury

16. Before beginning a primary survey, you should first—
    a. Position the victim so that you can open the airway.
    b. Call EMS professionals for help.
    c. Check for consciousness.
    d. Survey the scene.

17. Which first aid technique is used to provide oxygen to a victim of respiratory arrest?
    a. Cardiopulmonary resuscitation
    b. Oxygen supplementation by mask
    c. Rescue breathing
    d. Abdominal thrusts

18. Which must you do to determine if a victim requires rescue breathing?
    a. Look, listen, and feel for breathing.
    b. Check for a pulse in the neck.
    c. Check for bluish or grayish skin color.
    d. All of the above

19. How can you minimize the amount of air forced into a victim's stomach during rescue breathing?
    a. Do not pause between breaths unless absolutely necessary.
    b. Breathe slowly into the victim when delivering breaths.
    c. Press on the victim's stomach while delivering breaths.
    d. Breathe as hard as you can into the victim.

20. After discovering that your first two breaths are not causing the victim's chest to rise, what should you do?
    a. Retilt the head and give breaths again.
    b. Do a finger sweep.
    c. Give two more breaths with more force.
    d. Call EMS personnel.

21. When you give rescue breaths, how much air should you breathe into the victim?
    a. Enough to make the stomach rise
    b. Enough to make the chest rise
    c. Enough to feel resistance
    d. Enough to fill the victim's cheeks

22. What should you do for a conscious victim who is choking and cannot speak, cough, or breathe?
    a. Give abdominal thrusts.
    b. Give 2 full breaths.
    c. Do a finger sweep.
    d. Lower the victim to the floor and open the airway.

23. A woman is choking on a piece of candy, but is conscious and coughing forcefully. What should you do?
    a. Slap her on the back until she coughs up the object.
    b. Give abdominal thrusts.
    c. Encourage her to continue coughing.
    d. Do a finger sweep.

24. Which is your most important responsibility in caring for a victim complaining of shortness of breath and pressure in the chest?
    a. Having the victim stop what he is doing and rest in a comfortable position
    b. Providing CPR
    c. Asking the victim about previous medical conditions and helping him take nitroglycerine if prescribed
    d. Recognizing that these signals may indicate a heart attack.

25. Which should you do if a victim's breathing and heartbeat return while you are giving CPR?
    a. Keep the airway open and monitor vital signs until EMS personnel arrive.
    b. Have a bystander transport you and the victim to the nearest hospital.
    c. Complete a secondary survey before calling EMS personnel for assistance.
    d. Continue rescue breathing while waiting for EMS personnel to arrive.

26. High blood pressure can be controlled by—
    a. Changing dietary habits.
    b. Losing excess weight.
    c. Taking prescribed medication.
    d. All of the above

27. Which of the following is a risk factor for heart disease that cannot be controlled?
    a. High blood pressure
    b. Heredity
    c. Smoking
    d. Cholesterol level

28. The most prominent signal of a heart attack is—
    a. Profuse sweating.
    b. Pale skin.
    c. Persistent chest pain.
    d. Difficulty breathing.

29. CPR is needed—
    a. When the victim is not breathing.
    b. When the victim's heart stops beating.
    c. For every heart attack victim.
    d. When the heart attack victim loses consciousness.

30. The purpose of CPR is to—
    a. Keep a victim's airway open.
    b. Identify any immediate threats to life.
    c. Supply the vital organs with oxygen-rich blood.
    d. All of the above

31. How can you minimize the risk of disease transmission when controlling external bleeding?
    a. Use protective barriers such as gloves or plastic wrap.
    b. Minimize direct contact with blood.
    c. Wash your hands before and immediately after giving care.
    d. All of the above

32. What should you do if you suspect serious internal bleeding?
    a. Call EMS personnel immediately.
    b. Apply pressure at the closest pressure point.
    c. Place an ice pack on the affected area.
    d. Wrap a pressure bandage around the affected area.

33. Which signal is often the first indicator that the body is experiencing a problem that may result in shock?
    a. Nausea and vomiting
    b. Loss of consciousness
    c. Pale or bluish, cool, moist skin
    d. Restlessness or irritability

34. Which is the appropriate position for a victim who is showing the signals of shock as a result of injuries to the head and neck?
    a. Legs elevated about 24 inches
    b. Lying flat on the back
    c. Head and shoulders elevated about 12 inches
    d. On one side with head slightly elevated

35. The skin appears pale during shock as a result of—
    a. Constriction of blood vessels near the skin's surface.
    b. The majority of blood being sent to vital organs.
    c. Profuse sweating.
    d. a and b

36. Which would be part of your care for an infected wound?
    a. Cold, wet compresses
    b. Cold, dry compresses
    c. Hot, dry compresses
    d. Warm, wet compresses

37. Which factors affect the seriousness of a thermal burn?
    I. The temperature of the source of the burn
    II. The location of the burn on the body
    III. The sex of the individual burned
    IV. The extent of the burn
    V. The victim's age and medical condition

    ---

    a. All of the above
    b. I, II, IV, and V
    c. II, III, and IV
    d. II, III, and V

38. Signal(s) of infection include—
    a. Swelling or reddening around the wound.
    b. A throbbing pain.
    c. A cool sensation.
    d. a and b

39. When applying bandages—
    a. Cover the dressing completely.
    b. Cover fingers or toes.
    c. Remove any blood-soaked bandages and supply new ones.
    d. a and c

40. You should suspect a serious musculoskeletal injury if the victim tells you that she—
    a. Has a slight pain in her ankle when she walks.
    b. Has a history of frequent prior dislocations.
    c. Heard a snap or pop when she struck the ground.
    d. Notices that her injured wrist feels warm to the touch.

41. Which of the following are included in your general care for musculoskeletal injuries?
    a. Rest, ice, and elevation
    b. Ice and gentle exercise
    c. Splints, bandaging, and elevation
    d. Rest and heat packs

42. You should immobilize a musculoskeletal injury in order to—
    a. Prevent further soft tissue damage.
    b. Lessen pain.
    c. Lessen the danger of infection.
    d. All of the above

43. You would suspect a fracture or dislocation if—
    a. The victim could move the injured area without pain.
    b. The area was slightly swollen.
    c. The victim heard a snap at the time of the injury.
    d. a and b

44. For which of the following people should you consider the possibility of a serious head and/or spinal injury?
    a. A helmeted motorcyclist whose helmet was cracked as he hit the ground
    b. An 18-year-old who fell from a height of 3 feet
    c. A conscious victim of a motor vehicle crash who was not wearing a seat belt
    d. a and c

45. Which of the following is **not** a signal of head or spine injury?
    a. Elevated body temperature
    b. Partial or complete paralysis
    c. Confusion about the hour or day
    d. Tingling in the extremities

46. From which part of the body should you remove an impaled object if necessary to control bleeding?
    a. Chest
    b. Eye
    c. Cheek
    d. Hand

47. Which should be included in your basic care for serious chest or abdominal injuries?
    I. Calling EMS personnel
    II. Administering oxygen
    III. Applying ice or cold packs
    IV. Minimizing shock
    V. Limiting victim movement

    a. I, II, and IV
    b. I, IV, and V
    c. I, III, IV, and V
    d. II and V

48. Which position will a victim of a simple rib fracture often take?
    a. Sitting with a hand or arm supporting the chest
    b. Lying flat on the stomach
    c. Sitting with the shoulders back and chest out
    d. Lying flat on the back

49. Which signals indicate possible serious abdominal injury?
    I. Nausea and vomiting
    II. Respiratory distress
    III. Weakness and thirst
    IV. Coughing blood
    V. Bruising

    a. I and II
    b. III and IV
    c. I, III, and V
    d. II and III

50. In which position should you immobilize a suspected fracture or dislocation of the elbow?
    a. Slightly flexed with a rigid splint spanning and secured to the elbow
    b. Straight, immobilized with a rigid splint, and secured against the trunk
    c. Forearm supported in a sling and the upper arm secured to the body
    d. Any of the above, maintaining the position in which the elbow is found

51. Which of the following should be included in the immobilization of a suspected forearm fracture?

    I. A rigid splint secured from the site of the injury to the hand

    II. A roll of gauze or dressing material to keep the hand in a normal position

    III. A sling to support the forearm across the chest

    IV. Cravats to secure the arm to the victim's chest

    ---

    a. I and II

    b. I, III, and IV

    c. II, III, and IV

    d. IV

52. Which of the following are considered general signals of sudden illness?

    a. Change in level of consciousness

    b. Slowing pulse and breathing rates

    c. Nausea and vomiting

    d. All of the above

53. Your first aid care for a victim of fainting should include—

    I. Placing the victim in a semisitting position.

    II. Elevating the victim's legs.

    III. Giving a conscious victim small sips of water or fruit juice.

    IV. Conducting a primary survey.

    V. Splashing water on the victim's face.

    ---

    a. II and IV

    b. I, III, and V

    c. I and III

    d. II, IV, and V

54. Which should you include in your care for a conscious person who exhibits the signals of a diabetic emergency?

    a. Helping him or her to administer insulin.

    b. Giving sugar water or fruit juice to drink.

    c. Doing a secondary survey.

    d. b and c

55. A person in your office falls to the floor and begins to exhibit violent, uncontrolled movement. Which of the following first aid steps should you take?

I. Hold the person to protect him or her from injury.

II. Place a pillow or thick folded blanket under his or her head to protect it.

III. Place a pencil, ruler, or similar object between his or her teeth, if possible.

IV. Place the victim on his or her side when the seizure subsides.

V. Do a secondary survey following the seizure.

---

a. I, II, and IV

b. II, III, and V

c. IV and V

d. All of the above

56. Which of the following questions should you ask about a suspected poisoning to assist you in providing first aid?

I. Who was with the victim before the poisoning took place?

II. What type of poison was taken?

III. How much was taken?

IV. Does the victim have a history of drug abuse?

V. When was the poison taken?

VI. Has the victim been depressed or threatening suicide?

---

a. All of the above

b. I, II, IV, and VI

c. I and V

d. II, III, and V

57. When spending time outdoors in woods or tall grass, to prevent bites and stings you should—

a. Wear dark-colored clothing.

b. Wear loose-fitting clothing.

c. Tuck pant legs into boots or socks.

d. All of the above

58. In caring for an insect sting, you should—

a. Remove the remaining stinger by scraping it from the skin.

b. Remove the remaining stinger by using tweezers.

c. Wash the sting site, then cover it.

d. a and c

59. Which signals are you likely to observe in a person who has taken an overdose of depressants?
    a. Slurred speech, drowsiness, confusion
    b. Paranoia, rapid pulse, pinpoint pupils
    c. Sweating, chills, rapid pulse
    d. Euphoria, dry skin, flushed face

60. To avoid an unintentional misuse or overdose of a prescription drug, you should know the—
    a. Drugs with which it will interact.
    b. Effects of the drug.
    c. Potential side effects of the drug.
    d. All of the above

61. Which of the following is true of substance abuse?
    a. It is the use of a substance without regard to health concerns or accepted medical practices.
    b. It is the use of a substance for intended purposes but in improper amounts or doses.
    c. It occurs only among the elderly who are forgetful and may have poor eyesight.
    d. Its effects are minor and rarely result in medical complications.

62. As you are providing first aid to a victim of heat-related illness, which signals indicate that you should immediately call EMS personnel?
    a. The victim begins to sweat profusely.
    b. The victim loses consciousness.
    c. The victim refuses water or vomits.
    d. b and c

63. People who have taken certain types of substances are at increased risk of developing hypothermia. These substances include—
    a. Alcohol and barbiturates.
    b. Amphetamines and hallucinogens.
    c. Aspirin and diuretics.
    d. Caffeine and nicotine.

64. Precautions you can take that will help you prevent both heat- and cold-related illnesses include—
    a. Drinking plenty of fluids.
    b. Always wearing appropriate clothing for the environment.
    c. Keeping a constant, measured pace of activity while outdoors.
    d. a and b

65. If the victim of a suspected heat-related illness begins to lose consciousness, you should—
    a. Cool the body using wet sheets, towels, and cold packs.
    b. Cool the body by applying rubbing alcohol.
    c. Give cool water to drink.
    d. a and c

66. Which of the following should you consider to assure that you move a victim quickly and safely?
    a. Whether bystanders are available to help
    b. The size of the victim
    c. The victim's condition
    d. All of the above

67. In which of the following situations would you move a victim before providing first aid care?
    a. A victim lying in a supermarket aisle where a large crowd has gathered obstructing the aisle.
    b. A victim sitting in his truck on the shoulder of a busy highway; the truck's engine is running.
    c. A victim unconscious in his car in a closed garage; the car's engine is running.
    d. A victim who has fallen on her back in the bleachers at a high school football game; it is raining.

68. How does cardiovascular fitness contribute to a healthier lifestyle?
    a. It reduces the level of sugar in the blood.
    b. It helps to ward off infections.
    c. It improves individual self-esteem.
    d. b and c

69. To avoid reaching a level of blood alcohol that impairs judgment and reflexes, you should limit yourself to—
    a. One drink per hour.
    b. Two drinks per hour.
    c. Three drinks per hour.
    d. Four drinks per hour.

70. Which elements should you include in a fire escape plan for your home?
    a. Identification of at least two ways to get out of each room
    b. Designation of who will search each room before leaving the house
    c. Location of the phone from which the fire department will be called
    d. a and c

Answer Sheet: ARC First Aid—Responding to Emergencies

Name ____________________ Date ____________________ Exam ________

1.	a	b	c	d
2.	a	b	c	d
3.	a	b	c	d
4.	a	b	c	d
5.	a	b	c	d
6.	a	b	c	d
7.	a	b	c	d
8.	a	b	c	d
9.	a	b	c	d
10.	a	b	c	d
11.	a	b	c	d
12.	a	b	c	d
13.	a	b	c	d
14.	a	b	c	d
15.	a	b	c	d
16.	a	b	c	d
17.	a	b	c	d
18.	a	b	c	d
19.	a	b	c	d
20.	a	b	c	d
21.	a	b	c	d
22.	a	b	c	d
23.	a	b	c	d
24.	a	b	c	d
25.	a	b	c	d
26.	a	b	c	d
27.	a	b	c	d
28.	a	b	c	d
29.	a	b	c	d
30.	a	b	c	d
31.	a	b	c	d
32.	a	b	c	d
33.	a	b	c	d
34.	a	b	c	d
35.	a	b	c	d
36.	a	b	c	d
37.	a	b	c	d
38.	a	b	c	d
39.	a	b	c	d
40.	a	b	c	d
41.	a	b	c	d
42.	a	b	c	d
43.	a	b	c	d
44.	a	b	c	d
45.	a	b	c	d
46.	a	b	c	d
47.	a	b	c	d
48.	a	b	c	d
49.	a	b	c	d
50.	a	b	c	d
51.	a	b	c	d
52.	a	b	c	d
53.	a	b	c	d
54.	a	b	c	d
55.	a	b	c	d
56.	a	b	c	d
57.	a	b	c	d
58.	a	b	c	d
59.	a	b	c	d
60.	a	b	c	d
61.	a	b	c	d
62.	a	b	c	d
63.	a	b	c	d
64.	a	b	c	d
65.	a	b	c	d
66.	a	b	c	d
67.	a	b	c	d
68.	a	b	c	d
69.	a	b	c	d
70.	a	b	c	d

Appendix C

Test Bank Questions

This appendix contains approximately 500 questions. The number of questions for each textbook chapter is proportional to the amount of time spent on each subject during the course.

The questions are grouped according to the chapter and objective to which they relate. If a question is out of place, the appropriate objective is written above it.

The test bank includes multiple choice, matching, true/false, and short answer questions. In addition to being in bold type, the correct answers are indicated as follows:

Multiple choice	The correct answer is in bold type.
Matching	The correct answer is in front of the definition.
True/False	The correct answer is in brackets.
Short answer	Possible answers are listed.

The questions in the test bank may be used to prepare self-assessment exercises.

Except for two short answer questions (Chapter 4, Number 29 and Chapter 6, Number 7), all the questions in this appendix are included in the computerized test bank. As a result of the exclusion of these two questions—and a different way of numbering the matching questions—some of the question numbers are not identical to those in the computerized test bank.

The computerized test bank is available as a separate stock item. For the IBM version, order Stock No. 650022. For the Apple version, order Stock No. 650023.

Chapter 1—Introduction

Objective 1

1. Which of the following statements best describes the emergency medical services (EMS) system?

   a. The EMS system provides an ambulance to transport the victim to the hospital.

   b. The EMS system consists of community resources organized to care for victims of sudden illness or injury.

   c. Personnel and equipment for removing victims from dangerous locations are part of the EMS system.

   d. The EMS system is organized to prevent the occurrence of injuries and sudden illness.

2. Which individual in the EMS system provides the transition in care between the citizen responder level and medical professionals?

   a. EMS dispatcher

   b. First Responder

   c. Emergency medical technician

   d. Paramedic

Objective 2

3. The First Responder's role in the EMS system is identical to the role of the citizen responder.

   T—[F]

4. Which people in the EMS system have the role of recognizing that an emergency exists, deciding to act, activating the EMS system, and providing first aid?

   a. Paramedics

   b. Emergency medical technicians

   c. Firefighters

   d. Citizen responders

Objective 3

5. As a citizen responder, which is your most important responsibility in a life-threatening situation?

   a. Getting others to help you

   b. Summoning EMS professionals

   c. Moving the victim to safety

   d. Taking the victim to the hospital

6. When faced with a life-threatening emergency the most important action you can take as a citizen responder is to determine whether or not the victim is breathing and has a pulse.

   T—[F]

Objective 4

7. Unusual odors, sights, and noises are three of the common indicators of an emergency. What is the fourth?

   a. Unusual appearance or behavior

   b. Unexpected colors and lights

   c. Unusual arrangements of cars

   d. Unfamiliar organization of resources

Objective 5

8. Which of the following is a barrier to action in an emergency?

   a. Not wanting to get involved for fear of doing something wrong

   b. Uncertainty about providing first aid due to the nature of the injury or illness

   c. Embarrassment about stepping forward to provide first aid in front of strangers

   d. All of the above

9. If a victim's behavior threatens your safety while you are attempting to provide first aid, what should you do?

   a. Try to restrain the victim and prevent harm to yourself and others.

   b. Attempt to calm the victim by gently touching his or her arm and talking softly.

   c. Try speaking forcefully and authoritatively to the victim to gain cooperation.

   d. Withdraw from the immediate area and wait for EMS professionals.

10. Disease transmission from a victim to a rescuer requires four conditions. Which of the following is **not** one of the four?

    a. The victim must be infected with a disease.

    b. The rescuer providing first aid must be exposed to the infected victim's body fluids.

    c. The rescuer providing first aid must have bruises on the hands.

    d. There must be enough body fluids that contain germs to cause infection.

11. Citizen responders are infrequently sued.

[T]—F

12. Laws that protect people who willingly give first aid without accepting anything in return are called—

  a. Citizen responder laws.
  b. Hold Harmless laws.
  c. Good Samaritan laws.
  d. Medical Immunity laws.

Objective 6

13. The value of first aid training includes which of the following?

  a. A growth in confidence in responding to an emergency situation
  b. The knowledge of a plan of action useful in any emergency
  c. The development of skills that will help reduce family and personal medical cost
  d. a and b

14. Which of the following accurately describes the value of first aid training?

  a. It prepares you to provide medical treatment for the victim of an injury or sudden illness.
  b. It prepares you to confidently identify and manage most medical illnesses.
  c. It teaches you to prepare victims for transport to the hospital.
  d. It provides a basic plan of action that can be used in any emergency.

Objective 8

15. Match each term on the right with its definition on the left. Put its letter on the line in front of the definition.

f	An organization staffed by medical professionals trained to provide information about how to care for victims of poisoning	a.	Citizen responder
a	A layperson who recognizes an emergency and decides to help	b.	EMS dispatcher
c	A network of community resources and medical personnel that provides emergency care to victims of injury or sudden illness	c.	Emergency medical services (EMS) system
e	A person trained in emergency care called upon to provide such care as a routine part of his or her job	d.	Emergency operations center
		e.	First Responder
		f.	Poison Control Center

Objective 1

16. The role of the citizen responder includes—

  a. Recognizing that an emergency has occurred.
  b. Deciding to act.
  c. Providing advanced medical care.
  d. a and b

Chapter 2—Body Systems

Objective 1

1. The heart, blood, and blood vessels are major components of which body system?

  a. Nervous
  b. Integumentary
  c. Musculoskeletal
  d. Circulatory

2. Which structures of the musculoskeletal system usually join bone to bone at joints?

   a. Muscles
   b. Tendons
   c. Fibers
   d. Ligaments

3. Which structure listed below is part of the integumentary system?

   a. Muscle
   b. Skin
   c. Bone
   d. Nerves

Objective 2

4. In which structure of the respiratory system do oxygen and carbon dioxide pass in and out of the blood?

   a. Pharynx
   b. Trachea
   c. Bronchi
   d. Alveoli

5. Which system has primary responsibility for getting oxygen to each cell in the body?

   a. Nervous
   b. Circulatory
   c. Respiratory
   d. Integumentary

6. Which are the three primary functions of the nervous system?

   a. Sensory, motor, integrated
   b. Consciousness, memory, emotions
   c. Visual, olfactory, auditory
   d. Consciousness, regulation, language

7. Match each term on the right with its definition on the left. Put its letter on the line in front of the definition.

   b Group of organs that transports nutrients, oxygen, and wastes through the body

   a Group of organs that provides motion and strength

   d Group of organs that directs movement and sensory function

   c Group of organs that brings oxygen into the body and rids the body of carbon dioxide

   a. Musculoskeletal system
   b. Circulatory system
   c. Respiratory system
   d. Nervous system

Objective 3

8. In reaction to cold, the skin becomes pale and shows what is called "gooseflesh." Which two systems are interacting with the skin to maintain body temperature?

   a. Nervous, musculoskeletal
   b. Respiratory, integumentary
   c. Circulatory, musculoskeletal
   d. Nervous, circulatory

9. Which two body systems function with the alveoli to provide oxygen for the cells of the body?

   a. Musculoskeletal, integumentary
   b. Respiratory, circulatory
   c. Integumentary, respiratory
   d. Circulatory, musculoskeletal

10. The pain that accompanies a burn from hot water is an example of the interrelationship of which body systems?

    a. Respiratory, musculoskeletal
    b. Circulatory, respiratory
    c. Musculoskeletal, integumentary
    d. Integumentary, nervous

11. The respiratory system works with other body systems to provide oxygen to all body cells. These systems include the—

    a. Circulatory and nervous systems.
    b. Nervous system.
    c. Musculoskeletal, nervous, and circulatory systems.
    d. Musculoskeletal and circulatory systems.

12. The human body rapidly adapts to new environments. For example, when you step outside of an air-conditioned building on a hot, summer day, you immediately begin to sweat. Your body adapts to its "new" environment. What systems work together to produce this specific adaptation?

   a. Nervous and musculoskeletal systems
   b. Integumentary and respiratory systems
   c. Circulatory and respiratory systems
   d. Integumentary and nervous systems

Objective 4

13. Injuries to the musculoskeletal system may result in life-threatening damage to the circulatory and respiratory systems.

   [T]—F

Objective 5

14. Match each term on the right with its definition on the left. Put its letter on the line in front of the definition.

b	To breathe air out of the lungs	a.	Artery
a	Tube that carries blood away from the heart	b.	Exhale
d	Connecting structure between pharynx and bronchi	c.	Tissue
c	A collection of similar cells that performs a specific function	d.	Trachea

Chapter 3—Assessment

Objective 1

1. Which step of the emergency action principles should you take first?

   a. Doing a primary survey
   b. Doing a secondary survey
   c. Surveying the scene
   d. Calling EMS personnel for help

2. Before providing care for any victim, you should make sure the scene is safe for the victim and rescuers.

   [T]—F

3. The first thing you should do at any emergency scene is check victims for life-threatening conditions.

   T—[F]

Objective 2

4. Why should you follow the emergency action principles?

   a. They lead you to a diagnosis of the victim's illness or injury.
   b. They provide you with a detailed medical history of the victim.
   c. They ensure that necessary care is provided in any emergency.
   d. None of the above

5. Following the emergency action principles in every emergency will ensure your safety and the safety of others at the scene.

   [T]—F

6. When should you call EMS before doing a primary survey?

   a. When the victim is conscious
   b. When you suspect a poisonous gas is present
   c. When the emergency involves a child
   d. b and c

Objective 3

7. When you are already on the scene, when is it advisable to move a victim away from the scene before providing first aid?

   a. When the victim is complaining of being in an uncomfortable position
   b. When it is impossible to splint fractures or bandage wounds without moving the victim
   c. When the victim is in a position in which EMS personnel will have difficulty providing care
   d. When there is immediate danger such as poisonous fumes or an unstable structure

Objective 4

8. A car has crashed into a power pole and a live electrical wire is draped over its roof. The driver of the car is slumped against the steering wheel and appears to be bleeding heavily from a facial injury. What should be your immediate action in this situation?

   a. Approach the driver and determine if he is conscious and breathing.

   b. Move the live wire off the car using rubber gloves and a dry branch or pole.

   c. Instruct the driver to carefully open the door and jump clear of the car.

   d. Stay back from the car and call EMS personnel to deal with the situation.

9. You determine that a scene presents a dangerous situation and you cannot reach a victim to provide first aid. You should call EMS personnel and go to the nearest entrance to the scene to direct them to the victim.

   [T]—F

Objective 5

10. To which of these victims can you provide first aid because consent is implied?

    a. An unconscious victim

    b. An unaccompanied infant or child

    c. A victim unable to respond due to illness or injury

    d. All of the above

11. In addition to identifying yourself and your level of training to a conscious victim, what else must you tell the victim in order to obtain his or her consent to first aid care?

    a. Which ambulance service you are calling

    b. Where you received your training

    c. What you would like to do

    d. What you think is wrong with the victim

Objective 6

12. Why should you do a primary survey in every emergency situation?

    a. Because it protects you from legal liability

    b. Because it identifies conditions that are an immediate threat to life

    c. Because it identifies conditions that could become life-threatening if not cared for

    d. Because it enables you to protect the victim and bystanders from dangers at the scene

13. Why is it necessary to complete a primary survey in every emergency situation?

    a. To check for minor injuries

    b. To determine if there are any life-threatening conditions that need immediate care

    c. To get consent from the victim before providing care

    d. To ask for information about the cause of illness or injury

14. You should perform a primary survey on every victim because it identifies conditions that require immediate care.

    [T]—F

15. Performing a primary survey should take at least three minutes.

    T—[F]

Objective 7

16. A victim who can answer your question, "Are you O.K.?" is conscious and breathing and has a pulse.

    [T]—F

17. How should you determine if a victim is conscious?

    a. Slap the victim's face and ask, "Are you awake?"

    b. Pinch the muscle at the top of the victim's shoulder and ask, "Is this painful?"

    c. Gently tap the victim and ask, "Are you O.K.?"

    d. Rub your knuckles across the victim's sternum and ask, "Do you feel this?"

18. In what order do you assess the four elements of a primary survey? (first to last)

    a. Airway, breathing, circulation, consciousness
    b. Breathing, airway, circulation, consciousness
    c. Circulation, consciousness, airway, breathing
    d. Consciousness, airway, breathing, circulation

19. In the primary survey, checking circulation includes checking for a pulse, severe bleeding, and signs of shock.

    T—[F]

20. Before beginning a primary survey, you should first—

    a. Position the victim so that you can open the airway.
    b. Survey the scene.
    c. Check for consciousness.
    d. Call EMS professionals for help.

Objective 8

21. When calling EMS personnel for help, two things you tell the dispatcher are your name and the phone number from which you are calling.

    [T]—F

22. Once you have made a call for help to EMS personnel, you should hang up to keep the phone line clear.

    T—[F]

23. Which of the following questions is an EMS dispatcher likely to ask when you call for help?

    a. Who is the victim's doctor?
    b. Is first aid being given?
    c. Does the victim have allergies?
    d. Has the victim been drinking?

Objective 9

24. You should not call EMS personnel for help if the victim asks you not to.

    T—[F]

25. Your co-worker tells you that she has had pain in her abdomen for the past few hours and that it is suddenly much worse. You should call EMS personnel.

    [T]—F

26. You are walking with a neighbor when he steps off a curb and turns his ankle. He appears injured, but does not want you to call for help. After a few minutes, he wants to stand up. What should you do?

    a. Call EMS personnel; he may have a broken ankle.
    b. Get your car and drive him to the hospital.
    c. Help him stand up and reassess his condition.
    d. Call his doctor for advice.

27. For which of the following people should you **immediately** summon EMS personnel?

    a. A 22-year-old male who has had a fever and vomited twice during the night
    b. A 60-year-old jogger experiencing severe knee pain after a morning run
    c. A 40-year-old executive complaining that he has felt nauseated, sweaty, and short of breath for the past hour or so
    d. An 8-year-old with a large bruise on one arm from being hit by a baseball

Objective 10

28. When should you **not** perform a secondary survey?

    a. When caring for a conscious, cooperative victim
    b. When caring for a victim who has an obvious head injury
    c. When caring for a victim bleeding severely from the arm
    d. When caring for a victim complaining of pain in the neck and back

Objective 11

29. The purpose of the secondary survey is to—

    a. Find injuries or conditions that are not immediately life-threatening.
    b. Determine if the victim is bleeding severely.
    c. Survey the scene for hazardous conditions.
    d. Find out if the victim has medical insurance.

30. Which of the following conditions would you discover in a secondary survey?

    a. Cardiac arrest
    b. Open fracture with severe bleeding
    c. Allergies to bee stings and penicillin
    d. All of the above

31. You would discover changes in a victim's breathing and vital signs in the secondary survey.

    [T]—F

Objective 12

32. Which steps should you include in the secondary survey?

    a. Interviewing the victim and surveying the scene
    b. Sending a bystander to call EMS personnel and doing a head-to-toe examination
    c. Looking for hazards around the victim and checking for changes in the victim's breathing
    d. Doing a head-to-toe examination and interviewing bystanders

33. What information should you obtain in your interview of a victim?

    a. Age, address, next of kin
    b. Painful areas, allergies, current medications
    c. Name, age, religion
    d. What happened, medical conditions, vital signs

34. In performing a head-to-toe examination, you should ask the victim to carefully move any body part in which there is pain.

    T—[F]

35. Which technique would you **not** use to perform a head-to-toe examination of a victim?

    a. Visually inspecting the entire body, starting with the head
    b. Gently running your hands over each arm and leg to feel for possible fractures
    c. Asking the victim to take a deep breath and exhale, unless he or she previously complained of chest pain.
    d. Having the victim sit up if he or she can move all body parts without pain and has no apparent injuries

36. To which of the following should you give special attention during a secondary survey?

    a. Identification cards found in the victim's wallet
    b. A medical-alert bracelet
    c. The name and address of the victim's next of kin
    d. Cash and credit cards carried by the victim

Objective 13

37. Which victim might it be appropriate for you to transport to the hospital?

    a. A 42-year-old man complaining of chest pain that comes and goes
    b. A 10-year-old girl who fell from her bicycle and has an open fracture of the forearm
    c. A 50-year-old man whose hand was slammed in a door and is swollen and painful
    d. None of the above

38. You are alone with a victim whose condition you are certain is not severe. It would be appropriate for you to transport the victim to the hospital yourself as long as you watch for any changes in condition during the trip.

    T—[F]

Objective 14

39. If you decide to transport a victim to the hospital yourself, what precautions should you take?

    a. Have a bystander call the hospital and report the victim's condition.
    b. Make certain that the victim is transported lying down.
    c. Take a second person with you to ensure that the victim is constantly observed.
    d. Have a bystander notify the police to ask an officer to meet you at the hospital.

40. A victim's injuries appear to be minor. You should discourage him from driving to the hospital to be examined and treated.

    [T]—F

Objective 15

41. Match each term on the right with its definition on the left. Put its letter on the line in front of the definition.

d	Permission to provide care, given by the victim to the rescuer	a.	Primary survey
a	A check for immediate life-threatening conditions	b.	Emergency action principles
c	The status of a victim's breathing, pulse, and skin	c.	Vital signs
b	Steps that guide your actions as a citizen responder	d.	Consent

Chapter 4—Breathing Emergencies

Objective 1

1. A person in respiratory distress may appear to breathe more slowly than normal.

   [T]—F

2. Moist and flushed skin may signal respiratory distress.

   [T]—F

3. Which of the following is a signal of respiratory distress?

   a. Pain in the abdomen

   b. Tingling in the hands

   c. Constriction of the pupils

   d. None of the above

Objective 2

4. In which position should you always place a victim in respiratory distress?

   a. A sitting position

   b. Flat on the back

   c. On one side with the head down

   d. A position of comfort

5. If a victim of asthma has her prescribed medication available, you should assist her in taking it.

   [T]—F

6. If a victim is breathing, you do not need to check the pulse to determine whether the heart is beating.

   [T]—F

Objective 3

7. When you give rescue breathing, you are—

   a. Artificially circulating oxygen-rich blood to the body cells.

   b. Supplementing the air the victim is already breathing.

   c. Supplying the victim with oxygen necessary for survival.

   d. All of the above

8. Rescue breathing should be supplemented with added oxygen because exhaled air does not contain enough oxygen to sustain life.

   T—[F]

9. What percentage of the air you breathe out when giving rescue breathing is oxygen?

   a. 30 percent

   b. 21 percent

   c. 16 percent

   d. 12 percent

10. Which first aid technique is used to provide oxygen to a victim of respiratory arrest?

    a. Cardiopulmonary resuscitation

    b. Oxygen supplementation by mask

    c. Rescue breathing

    d. Abdominal thrusts

Objective 4

11. Rescue breathing alone will be of benefit to a victim whose heart has stopped beating.

    T—[F]

12. For which condition should you give rescue breathing?

    a. Respiratory distress
    b. Cardiac arrest
    c. Asthma
    d. Respiratory arrest

13. During which emergency action step will you determine if a victim requires rescue breathing?

    a. Secondary survey
    b. Survey of the scene
    c. Primary survey
    d. Preparation for transport

14. Which must you do to determine if a victim requires rescue breathing?

    a. Check for a pulse in the neck.
    b. Look, listen, and feel for breathing.
    c. Check for bluish or grayish skin color.
    d. All of the above

15. A victim who has a pulse does not require rescue breathing.

    T—[F]

Objective 5

16. You have decided to give rescue breathing to a victim of respiratory arrest. Which technique should you use to keep the airway open?

    a. Chin lift
    b. Head-tilt/neck-lift
    c. Modified jaw thrust
    d. Head-tilt/chin-lift

17. Which is the most dependable method of evaluating the effectiveness of rescue breathing?

    a. Assuring that your mouth is sealed securely against the victim's mouth
    b. Assuring that the victim's nose is pinched securely shut
    c. Breathing into the victim's mouth for exactly 1 to $1^1/_2$ seconds
    d. Seeing the victim's chest rise with each breath you deliver

18. If the victim's head is not tilted enough when you deliver breaths during rescue breathing, what will happen?

    a. Air may go into the victim's stomach.
    b. Oxygen will not get to the victim's tissues.
    c. No air will go into the victim's lungs.
    d. The victim's pharynx will rupture.

19. How can you minimize the amount of air forced into a victim's stomach during rescue breathing?

    a. Breathe slowly into the victim when delivering breaths.
    b. Do not pause between breaths unless absolutely necessary.
    c. Press on the victim's stomach while delivering breaths.
    d. Breathe as hard as you can into the victim.

20. Breathing into a victim for longer than 1 to $1^1/_2$ seconds per breath can cause gastric distention.

    [T]—F

21. Gastric distention rarely causes vomiting during rescue breathing.

    T—[F]

22. When you give rescue breaths, how much air should you breathe into the victim?

    a. Enough to make the stomach rise
    b. Enough to make the chest rise
    c. Enough to feel resistance
    d. Enough to fill the victim's cheeks

23. Assuring adequate head-tilt, breathing slowly into the victim's mouth, and stopping the breath when the victim's chest rises will help avoid getting air into the victim's stomach during rescue breathing.

    [T]—F

24. When performing rescue breathing, what should you do after giving the first 2 full breaths?

    a. Adjust the head-tilt to a neutral position and continue rescue breathing.
    b. Check for a pulse; if present, continue rescue breathing.
    c. Continue rescue breathing if the victim has no heartbeat.
    d. Call for help from EMS professionals.

25. You should check the victim for a pulse every minute while providing rescue breathing.

[T]—F

26. If a victim has dentures, you should remove them before starting rescue breathing.

T—[F]

Objective 6

27. Trying to swallow large pieces of food is a common cause of choking.

[T]—F

28. Drinking alcohol with meals helps people relax and reduces the risk of choking.

T—[F]

29. List three causes of choking:

____

____

____

1. **Trying to swallow large pieces of food**
2. **Drinking alcohol before or during meals**
3. **Eating while talking excitedly or laughing, or eating too fast**
4. **Wearing dentures**
5. **Walking, playing, or running with food or objects in the mouth**

Objective 7

30. If you are alone and choking, you are going to die because you cannot help yourself.

T—[F]

31. By leaning forward and pressing his or her abdomen over a chair back, railing, or kitchen cabinet, a choking victim can give himself or herself abdominal thrusts.

[T]—F

32. Which is the first step you should take to aid an unconscious choking victim?

a. Place one fist on the victim's abdomen just above the navel, well below the sternum.

b. Give quick, upward thrusts into the abdomen.

c. Straddle one or both of the victim's thighs.

d. Call EMS personnel.

33. After discovering that your first 2 breaths are not causing the victim's chest to rise, what should you do?

a. Call EMS personnel.

b. Do a finger sweep.

c. Give 2 more breaths with more force.

d. Retilt the head and give breaths again.

34. What should you do for a conscious victim who is choking and cannot speak, cough, or breathe?

a. Give abdominal thrusts.

b. Give 2 full breaths.

c. Do a finger sweep.

d. Lower the victim to the floor and open the airway.

35. After giving your first series of 6 to 10 abdominal thrusts to an unconscious victim with an obstructed airway, you should—

a. Do a finger sweep and then give 2 full breaths.

b. Give 2 full breaths and then do a finger sweep.

c. Check for pulse, give 2 full breaths, and do a finger sweep.

d. Do a finger sweep and check for pulse.

36. While eating dinner, a friend suddenly starts to cough weakly and make high-pitched noises. You should—

a. Lower him to the floor, do a finger sweep, give 2 full breaths and 6 to 10 abdominal thrusts.

b. Give abdominal thrusts until the object is dislodged or he becomes unconscious.

c. Encourage him to continue coughing to try to dislodge the object.

d. Open the airway using the head-tilt/chin-lift.

37. A woman is choking on a piece of candy but is conscious and coughing forcefully. What should you do?

a. Slap her on the back until she coughs up the object.

b. Give abdominal thrusts.

c. Encourage her to continue coughing.

d. Do a finger sweep.

Chapter 5—Cardiac Emergencies

Objective 1

1. The most prominent signal of a heart attack is—

   a. Profuse sweating.

   b. Pale skin.

   c. Persistent chest pain.

   d. Difficulty breathing.

2. Brief, stabbing chest pains are signals of a heart attack.

   T—[F]

3. Chest pain that worsens when the victim breathes deeply is frequently a sign of a heart attack.

   T—[F]

4. Some victims of a heart attack experience no chest pain.

   [T]—F

5. Which is the key signal of a heart attack?

   a. Difficulty breathing

   b. Pain in the jaw and left arm

   c. Nausea and sweating

   d. Persistent chest pain

6. For the citizen responder, which difference between heart attack and angina pectoris is most important?

   a. Angina attacks last less than 10 minutes; heart attack pain goes on for several hours.

   b. Angina pain is "sharp"; heart attack pain is "crushing."

   c. Angina pain usually decreases when the victim rests and takes his or her medication; heart attack pain does not.

   d. All of the above

7. Why are the coronary arteries important?

   a. They supply oxygen-rich blood to the head.

   b. They transport blood to the lungs, where it receives new oxygen.

   c. They supply oxygen-rich blood to the heart muscle.

   d. They contain sensors that regulate heart rate.

Objective 2

8. Which is your most important responsibility in caring for a victim complaining of shortness of breath and pressure in the chest?

   a. Having the victim stop what he is doing and rest in a comfortable position

   b. Providing CPR

   c. Asking the victim about previous medical conditions and helping him take nitroglycerine if prescribed

   d. Recognizing that these signals may indicate a heart attack

9. Caring for a heart attack victim may include going against the victim's wishes.

   [T]—F

10. In which position should you place a victim who may be experiencing a heart attack?

    a. Lying on the left side

    b. Sitting or semisitting

    c. The most comfortable position

    d. Lying on the back with legs elevated

11. You should not assist a victim complaining of chest pain in taking his prescribed nitroglycerine.

    T—[F]

12. If you suspect a victim is having a heart attack, it may be better for you to drive the victim to the hospital yourself to save time rather than wait for EMS personnel.

    T—[F]

Objective 3

13. Which is the most common cause of cardiac arrest?

    a. Electrocution

    b. Drowning/suffocation

    c. Cardiovascular disease

    d. Drug overdose/poisoning

14. A victim is described as being clinically dead. What has happened?

    a. Breathing has stopped.

    b. Blood pressure is too low to measure.

    c. Breathing and heartbeat have stopped.

    d. The victim has sustained brain damage.

15. Which is the primary signal of cardiac arrest?

    a. Absence of a radial pulse
    b. No breathing
    c. Dilation of the pupils
    d. Absence of a carotid pulse

Objective 4

16. Which is the purpose of cardiopulmonary resuscitation (CPR)?

    a. To restart heartbeat and breathing in a victim of cardiac arrest
    b. To keep the brain supplied with oxygen until the heart can be restarted
    c. To prevent clinical death from occurring in a victim of cardiac arrest
    d. All of the above

17. CPR is needed—

    a. When the victim is not breathing.
    b. When the victim's heart stops beating.
    c. For every heart attack victim.
    d. When the heart attack victim loses consciousness.

18. The purpose of CPR is to—

    a. Keep a victim's airway open.
    b. Identify any immediate threats to life.
    c. Supply the vital organs with oxygen-rich blood.
    d. All of the above

19. If CPR is not started, how long after cardiac arrest will the brain begin to die?

    a. Immediately
    b. 2 to 4 minutes
    c. 4 to 6 minutes
    d. 8 to 10 minutes

20. The point at which the brain sustains irreversible damage due to brain cell death from lack of oxygen is called—

    a. Biological death.
    b. Cardiac arrest.
    c. Clinical death.
    d. Statutory death.

21. Calling EMS personnel promptly is important in cases of cardiac arrest. This is because even well-performed CPR generates only about one third of the normal blood flow to the brain, and advanced medical care is needed for resuscitation.

    [T]—F

22. If CPR is started within 6 minutes of a cardiac arrest and is properly performed, approximately 75 percent of victims survive to be discharged from the hospital.

    T—[F]

Objective 5

23. Your first action in caring for a victim who may have sustained a cardiac arrest is to—

    a. Find the correct hand position on the chest for compressions.
    b. Call EMS personnel.
    c. Perform a primary survey.
    d. Ask bystanders how long the victim has been ill or injured.

24. Which is the correct hand position for delivering chest compressions to an adult?

    a. Over the xiphoid process
    b. Over the lower half of the sternum
    c. Over the middle of the sternum
    d. Just below the notch where the ribs meet the sternum

25. A citizen responder who suffers from arthritis or a similar condition may perform CPR by grasping the wrist of the hand on the victim's chest with his or her other hand.

    [T]—F

26. Which cadence should you use when counting aloud during cardiac compressions on an adult victim?

    a. "One one thousand, two one thousand, ..." up to 15
    b. "One, two, three, four, ..." up to 15
    c. "One and two and three and four ..." up to 15
    d. Any of the above is acceptable.

27. Once you have started CPR, when should you check to determine whether the victim has a pulse?

    a. After the first two minutes (eight cycles) and every two minutes thereafter

    b. After the first minute (four cycles) and every few minutes thereafter

    c. After each minute (four cycles) of continuous CPR

    d. Any of the above is acceptable.

28. You are aiding a person who may be a victim of cardiac arrest. No one has responded to your shouts for help. At which point in your efforts should you call for EMS personnel?

    a. Before you begin rescue breathing

    b. As soon as you determine that there is no carotid pulse

    c. After delivering one minute of continuous CPR

    d. When you become exhausted and need to rest

29. If two rescuers trained in CPR are at the scene of a cardiac arrest, they should share the CPR efforts. One rescuer should deliver the chest compressions and the other do the rescue breathing.

    T—[F]

Objective 6

30. When should you stop providing CPR?

    I. When EMS personnel take over

    II. When a neighbor tells you to stop

    III. When you are exhausted

    IV. If the scene becomes unsafe

    V. If the victim vomits

    ---

    a. I, III, and IV

    b. II and IV

    c. V only

    d. All of the above

31. Which should you do if another trained person takes over CPR from you?

    a. Assist by checking the carotid pulse for an artificial pulse during compressions.

    b. Call EMS personnel if this has not been done.

    c. Make certain the victim's chest rises and falls during rescue breathing.

    d. All of the above

32. Which should you do if a victim's breathing and heartbeat return while you are giving CPR?

    a. Continue rescue breathing while waiting for EMS personnel to arrive.

    b. Have a bystander transport you and the victim to the nearest hospital.

    c. Complete a secondary survey before calling EMS personnel for assistance.

    d. Keep the airway open and monitor vital signs until EMS personnel arrive.

Objective 7

33. A person quits smoking after having smoked for 15 years. Over time, his risk of heart attack from his smoking will decline until he is at no greater risk of a heart attack than a person who has never smoked.

    [T]—F

34. High blood pressure can be controlled by—

    a. Losing excess weight.

    b. Taking prescribed medication.

    c. Changing dietary habits.

    d. All of the above

35. How can you decrease the amount of saturated fats in your diet?

    a. Use cholesterol-free products in cooking.

    b. Substitute skim milk for whole milk.

    c. Eat lamb instead of beef.

    d. All of the above

36. How much greater risk of a fatal heart attack do overweight middle-aged men have than normal-weight men of similar age?

    a. Twice the risk

    b. Three times the risk

    c. Four times the risk

    d. Six times the risk

37. There is no need for a low-fat diet when routine exercise alone has been shown to decrease the incidence of heart attacks.

    T—[F]

38. Which of the following is a risk factor for heart disease that cannot be controlled?

a. High blood pressure

b. Heredity

c. Smoking

d. Cholesterol level

Objective 8

39. Match each term on the right with its definition on the left. Put its letter on the line in front of the definition.

g	A sudden illness involving death of heart muscle tissue due to insufficient oxygen-rich blood reaching the cells	a.	Angina pectoris
c	A technique combining rescue breathing with chest compressions	b.	Cardiac arrest
d	A chronic illness affecting the heart and blood vessels	c.	Cardiopulmonary resuscitation
f	A device that sends an electrical shock through the heart to enable a heart that has stopped circulating blood to resume a normal heartbeat	d.	Cardiovascular disease
h	An arrow-shaped piece of hard tissue at the lowest point of the sternum	e.	Cartilage
b	A condition in which the heart has stopped or beats too irregularly or weakly to pump blood effectively	f.	Defibrillator
		g.	Heart attack
		h.	Xiphoid

Chapter 6—Bleeding

Objective 1

Check the true statements. Correct the false statements to make them true.

❑ **1. Blood consists of liquid and solid components.**

❑ **2. A key disease-fighting part of the immune system is in the blood.**

❑ 3. White blood cells are produced in the marrow of large bones. (Incorrect—Red blood cells are produced in the marrow of large bones.)

❑ **4. Plasma makes up about one-half of the total blood volume.**

5. Why might severe bleeding result in death?

a. The supply of necessary nutrients to the heart is reduced.

b. Decreased blood volume deprives body tissues of oxygen.

c. Blood vessels collapse as blood volume decreases.

d. Vital disease-fighting components are lost with the blood.

6. Which is one of the major functions of blood?

a. Transporting nutrients and oxygen

b. Carrying minerals to bones

c. Maintaining pressure within blood vessels

d. Preventing internal bleeding

Objective 2

7. List three major functions of blood.

____

____

____

1. Transporting oxygen, nutrients, and wastes

2. Protecting against disease by producing antibodies and defending against germs

3. Maintaining constant body temperature by circulating throughout the body

Objective 3

8. Only external bleeding that spurts from a wound is potentially life-threatening.

T—[F]

9. External bleeding is not usually an emergency.

 [T]—F

Objective 4

10. When trying to control external bleeding, leave blood-soaked dressings in place.

 [T]—F

11. Which is the first step in managing external bleeding?
 a. Add bulky dressings to reinforce blood-soaked bandages.
 b. Apply pressure at a pressure point.
 c. Apply direct pressure with a clean or sterile pad.
 d. Apply a pressure bandage.

Objective 5

12. How can you minimize the risk of disease transmission when controlling external bleeding?
 a. Wash your hands before and immediately after giving care.
 b. Minimize direct contact with blood.
 c. Use protective barriers such as gloves or plastic wrap.
 d. All of the above

Objective 6

13. Nausea and vomiting, decreasing level of consciousness, and pale or bluish sweaty skin are signals of which of the following conditions?
 a. Internal bleeding
 b. Heat stroke
 c. Stimulant overdose
 d. Frostbite

Objective 7

14. Five signals of internal bleeding are—rapid, weak pulse; rapid breathing; nausea and vomiting; excessive thirst; and discoloration of skin in injured area.

 [T]—F

15. You can control serious internal bleeding by applying ice packs to the injured area.

 T—[F]

16. What should you do for a victim who appears to have serious internal bleeding?
 a. Apply heat to the injured area.
 b. Place the victim in a sitting position.
 c. Give fluids to drink to replace blood loss.
 d. Call EMS personnel.

17. What should you do if you suspect serious internal bleeding?
 a. Call EMS personnel immediately.
 b. Apply pressure at the closest pressure point.
 c. Place an ice pack on the affected area.
 d. Wrap a pressure bandage around the affected area.

18. Internal bleeding resulting from violent blunt force is almost always an emergency.

 [T]—F

19. You and a friend are the first persons to arrive at the scene of a single car crash. The driver has gotten out of the vehicle without assistance and is sitting on the ground near the road. You see no blood or other obvious injuries. He is complaining of pain in his abdomen. He also complains of nausea.
 When you look under his shirt, you see that the skin across the lower abdomen is beginning to show bruising. Match the following actions with the order in which you would perform them.

 d First action
 c Second action
 a Third action

 a. Monitor the ABCs.
 b. Walk the victim to your car.
 c. Provide care to prevent or minimize shock.
 d. Have your friend call EMS personnel.

Objective 8

20. Which term is used to denote a site on the body where pressure can be applied to a major artery to slow the flow of blood to a body part?
 a. Control point
 b. Arterial point
 c. Pressure point
 d. Stress point

21. Which term describes the loss of a large amount of blood in a short period of time?

   a. Internal bleeding
   b. Hemorrhage
   c. Capillary bleeding
   d. Evisceration

Chapter 7—Shock

Objective 1

1. Shock is a condition resulting only from severe blood loss.

   T—[F]

2. Which can cause a victim to develop shock?

   a. Severe blood loss
   b. Smoke inhalation
   c. Injury to the spinal cord
   d. All of the above

3. A person who is injured and very frightened is less likely to develop shock than one who is calm.

   T—[F]

Objective 2

4. Which signal is often the first indicator that the body is experiencing a problem that may result in shock?

   a. Nausea and vomiting
   b. Loss of consciousness
   c. Restlessness or irritability
   d. Pale or bluish, cool, moist skin

5. Why does the skin of a victim in shock appear pale and feel cool?

   a. Because shock damages the temperature control centers in the brain and spinal cord
   b. Because the body responds to shock by reducing the amount of blood going to the skin
   c. Because shock causes the heart to slow, reducing the amount of heat generated by the body
   d. Because the body responds to shock by cooling itself to decrease energy needs

6. Which signal of shock results from a prolonged lack of oxygen?

   a. Excessive thirst
   b. Nausea and vomiting
   c. Pale, moist skin
   d. Bluish-tinged lips

7. The skin appears pale during shock as a result of—

   a. Constriction of blood vessels near the skin's surface.
   b. The majority of blood being sent to vital organs.
   c. Profuse sweating.
   d. a and b

Objective 3

8. Which of the following measures would minimize shock?

   a. Reducing the victim's body temperature
   b. Raising the victim's body temperature
   c. Maintaining the victim's normal body temperature
   d. Allowing the victim's body temperature to regulate itself

9. A victim of serious injury complains of extreme thirst. You should give him a few sips of water to help to minimize shock.

   T—[F]

10. Which is the appropriate position for a victim who is showing the signals of shock as a result of injuries to the head and neck?

   a. Legs elevated about 24 inches
   b. Head and shoulders elevated about 12 inches
   c. Lying flat on the back
   d. On one side with head slightly elevated

11. Wait to give care to minimize shock until you have completed a secondary survey.

   T—[F]

Objective 4

12. Match each term on the right with its definition on the left. Put its letter on the line in front of the definition.

e	Failure of the circulatory system to provide adequate oxygen-rich blood to all parts of the body	a.	Blood volume
b	Bluish tinge of the lips, eyelids, and nailbeds resulting from prolonged lack of oxygen	b.	Cyanosis
a	The total amount of blood circulating within the body	c.	Injury
d	Sudden illness resulting from problems within the body	d.	Medical emergency
		e.	Shock

Chapter 8—Soft Tissue Injuries

Objective 1

1. Which skin layer contains nerves, oil glands, and blood vessels?

   a. Epidermis

   b. Dermis

   c. Subcutaneous

   d. Fatty

2. Which signals indicate that a victim has a closed wound of the thigh?

   a. A trickle of blood on the thigh; the victim complains of thigh pain

   b. A painful white lump on the thigh

   c. A raised dark red area on the thigh

   d. A wide reddened area on the thigh covered with tiny droplets of blood

Objective 2

3. Two of the main dangers associated with open wounds are severe bleeding and infection.

   [T]—F

4. Which type of wound carries the greatest risk of tetanus infection?

   a. Abrasion

   b. Laceration

   c. Avulsion

   d. Puncture

5. Which should you do to minimize the risk of infection in a minor abrasion on a child's arm?

   a. Wash the abrasion with soap and water.

   b. Cover the area with several dressings.

   c. Take the child to a doctor for a tetanus booster.

   d. All of the above

6. Before applying a dressing and direct pressure, you should let a large laceration bleed for a few seconds to minimize the risk of infection.

   T—[F]

7. How often should you receive a tetanus booster if you are under 65?

   a. Every 2 years

   b. Every 3 to 5 years

   c. Every 5 to 10 years

   d. Every 10 to 15 years

Objective 3

8. Which of the following signals indicates that a wound in the palm of the hand is infected?

   I. Tingling in the fingertips

   II. Redness and warmth in the palm

   III. Stiffness in the elbow

   IV. Throbbing pain in the palm and wrist

   V. Red streaks on the inner forearm

   VI. Bluish tinge to the nail beds

   ---

   a. All of the above

   b. III, IV, and V

   c. II, IV, and V

   d. I, II, and VI

9. About a week after the sole of your left foot is lacerated, you notice the foot is swollen and sore. The wound area looks red and the wound is oozing a small amount of yellow fluid. Which of the following conclusions would you draw?

   a. The wound is healing normally
   b. The wound may require stitches
   c. A foot bone may be fractured
   d. The wound has become infected

10. Signals of infection include—

   a. Swelling or reddening around the wound.
   b. A throbbing pain.
   c. A cool sensation.
   d. a and b

Objective 4

11. Caring for an infected wound includes—

   a. Keeping the area uncovered.
   b. Seeking medical help if the infection persists.
   c. Applying cool wet compresses.
   d. All of the above

12. Which would be part of your care for an infected wound?

   a. Cold, wet compresses
   b. Cold, dry compresses
   c. Hot, dry compresses
   d. Warm, wet compresses

13. Which should you do if a person who has sustained an open wound develops a fever and you see red streaks toward the heart from the wound?

   a. Apply an antibiotic ointment to the wound.
   b. Seek medical care without delay.
   c. Wash the wound and elevate the area.
   d. Change the dressing and apply cold compresses.

Objective 5

14. The purposes of a bandage include—

   a. Holding a dressing in place and providing support to injured body parts.
   b. Keeping air from an open wound and keeping a wound warm.
   c. Providing pressure to help control bleeding, and protecting a wound from infection.
   d. a and c

15. The difference between a dressing and a bandage is that dressings are applied directly over an open wound and bandages are used to hold dressings in place.

   [T]—F

16. Which of the following guidelines should you follow when applying a bandage?

   I. Leave a corner of the dressing exposed to check it for blood saturation.
   II. Elevate the injured part above the level of the heart, if safe to do so.
   III. Do not cover the fingers or toes unless absolutely necessary.
   IV. Remove and replace a dressing that becomes saturated with blood.
   V. Loosen the bandage slightly if fingers or toes below the bandage become pale.

   ---

   a. All of the above
   b. I and IV
   c. II, III, IV, and V
   d. II, III, and V

Objective 6

17. When applying bandages—

   a. Cover the dressing completely.
   b. Cover fingers or toes.
   c. Remove any blood-soaked bandages and apply new ones.
   d. a and c

18. Which is the proper first aid care for a closed wound?

   a. Massage and dry, warm packs
   b. Direct pressure, elevation, and cold
   c. Elastic bandage and range of motion exercise
   d. Rest, aspirin, and vitamin C

19. When a body part is completely severed, bleeding is usually so severe that applying pressure to a pressure point is needed to control it.

   T—[F]

20. A driver sustained a closed wound of the thigh in an automobile crash. It is unlikely that he will require transportation to a hospital.

   T—[F]

21. If no sterile dressing is available to place over a severely bleeding wound, the next best thing to use to control the bleeding is your bare hand.

    T—[F]

22. Which should be part of your care for a severely bleeding open wound?

    a. Washing the wound and covering it with a sterile dressing

    b. Elevating the body part and applying direct pressure

    c. Washing your hands after completing care

    d. b and c

23. Which should be included in first aid care for a victim whose finger has been severed?

    a. Placing the severed finger directly in a container of cold or ice water

    b. Wrapping the finger in a clean dressing, placing it in a plastic bag, and keeping the bag on ice

    c. Wrapping the finger in sterile gauze and keeping it warm and dry

    d. Placing the unwrapped finger in a plastic bag and keeping the bag on ice

24. You are unable to stop the bleeding around a piece of broken glass impaled in a victim's upper arm by using bulky dressings and pressure around the glass. You should carefully remove the glass and apply direct pressure to the wound.

    T—[F]

25. Which should be included in your first aid care for a wound with minimal bleeding and superficial damage?

    a. Washing the wound with soap and water before controlling bleeding

    b. After bleeding is stopped, applying an antibiotic ointment

    c. Applying a sterile dressing over the wound and then a bandage

    d. All of the above

***Objective** 7*

26. Which is the most common type of burn?

    a. Chemical

    b. Lightning

    c. Heat

    d. Solar radiation

27. The most common cause of burn injuries is exposure to corrosive chemicals.

    T—[F]

Objective 8

28. What would you take into account in evaluating the severity of a burn?

    a. The number of victims burned

    b. The age and health status of the victim

    c. The amount and type of clothing the victim was wearing

    d. The time of day the burn was acquired

29. Which factors affect the seriousness of a thermal burn?

    I. The temperature of the source of the burn

    II. The location of the burn on the body

    III. The gender of the individual burned

    IV. The extent of the burn

    V. The victim's age and medical condition

    ---

    a. All of the above

    b. I, II, IV, and V

    c. II, III, and IV

    d. II, III, and V

30. Which signals would indicate that a person has a superficial burn?

    a. The skin is red, dry, and painful.

    b. The skin is pale, wet, and painful.

    c. The skin is red, wet, and painless.

    d. The skin is mottled, dry, and painless.

31. Which type of burn results in skin that is red, weeps clear fluid, and is painful and swollen?

    a. Superficial burn

    b. Partial-thickness burn

    c. Full-thickness burn

    d. Mixed-thickness burn

32. When a burn appears brown or charred, shows white tissue underneath, and is almost painless, what has been injured?

    a. The epidermis

    b. The epidermis and dermis

    c. The epidermis, dermis, and fatty tissues

    d. The epidermis, dermis, and underlying soft tissue structures

33. In many cases, full-thickness burns are less likely to cause shock than partial-thickness burns because they are often painless, where as partial-thickness burns cause severe pain.

T—[F]

Objective 9

34. The severity of pain felt by the victim of a burn increases as the severity of the burn increases.

T—[F]

35. In which of the following situations should you immediately call EMS personnel?

a. A partial-thickness burn to a child's forearm

b. A chemical burn to an adult's lower leg

c. A superficial burn to a teenager's hand

d. a and b

36. In which of the following situations should you immediately call EMS personnel?

a. A partial-thickness water scald to the right upper arm of a 30-year-old man

b. A blistered grease burn on the hands and arms of a 68-year-old woman

c. A sunburn to the back of a 26-year-old woman

d. a and b

37. You should immediately call EMS personnel for burns resulting from a chemical, an explosion, or electricity.

[T]—F

Objective 10

38. Which is your first consideration in a situation in which a person has been seriously burned?

a. Completing a primary survey

b. Surveying the scene for safety

c. Calling EMS personnel

d. Cooling the burned area

39. How should you cool a partial-thickness thermal burn?

a. Strip away burned clothing.

b. Gently fan the victim with a towel.

c. Use ice packs or ice water.

d. Use large amounts of cool water.

40. You have cooled a full-thickness thermal burn. Which step should you take next in your first aid care?

a. Remove any clothing sticking to the skin.

b. Apply a commercial burn ointment, if available.

c. Cover with a sterile dressing and bandage loosely.

d. Place an airtight dressing over the burn and bandage.

41. A person who has sustained a full-thickness burn may develop the signals of shock from loss of body fluids through the burn.

[T]—F

42. Burns that require professional medical attention—

a. Are only those that affect the limbs.

b. Are those resulting from electricity, explosions, or chemicals.

c. Are burns whose victims are having difficulty breathing.

d. b and c

Objective 11

43. Your sister has accidentally splashed floor cleaner into her eyes. What should you do?

a. Flush her eyes with warm water for at least 10 minutes.

b. Flush her eyes with vinegar and water to neutralize the chemical.

c. Flush her eyes with tap water until EMS personnel arrive.

d. Flush her eyes with water for 2 to 3 minutes and call EMS personnel.

44. In caring for the victim of an electrical injury, you should—

a. Push the victim away from any electrical wires with a dry pole or stick.

b. Look for an entrance and exit wound.

c. Cover any burn with a dry, sterile dressing.

d. b and c

45. A victim of a lightning strike should be moved as quickly as possible inside a building or automobile for protection against further strikes.

T—[F]

46. First aid care for a partial-thickness sunburn should include application of ointments made specially to reduce the effects of sunburn.

T—[F]

Objective 12

47. Match each term on the right with its definition on the left. Put its letter on the line in front of the definition.

b	Material placed directly over a wound to absorb blood and prevent infection	a.	Bandage
c	An injury involving all layers of skin and underlying tissues	b.	Dressing
f	An injury involving only the epidermis	c.	Full-thickness burn
a	Material used to hold a splint or a sterile wound covering in place	d.	Open wound
		e.	Partial-thickness burn
		f.	Superficial burn

Chapter 9—Musculoskeletal Injuries

Objective 1

1. Which type of muscle provides for movement of the body?

   a. Involuntary muscle

   b. Skeletal muscle

   c. Cardiac muscle

   d. All of the above

2. Which of the following structures make up the musculoskeletal system?

   I. Muscles

   II. Bones

   III. Skin

   IV. Tendons

   V. Ligaments

   a. I and II

   b. II, III, and IV

   c. I, II, IV, and V

   d. I, IV, and V

3. Muscles are attached to bones by strong, cordlike tissues called ligaments.

   T–[F]

4. Which of the following is an irregular bone?

   a. Upper arm

   b. Sternum

   c. Shoulder blade

   d. Vertebra

5. Joints are held together by tough, fibrous connective tissues called tendons.

   T—[F]

Objective 2

6. A fracture of the radius caused by a bullet entering the arm is an open fracture.

   [T]—F

7. Before an injury can be called a sprain, what must be injured?

   a. A tendon

   b. A ligament

   c. Cartilage

   d. All of the above

8. Injuries to the musculoskeletal system are identified and cared for during the—

   a. Secondary survey.

   b. Primary survey.

   c. ABCs.

   d. Survey of the scene.

9. In which of the following musculoskeletal injuries is there usually no apparent deformity?

   a. Fracture

   b. Dislocation

   c. Strain

   d. All of the above

10. The amount of swelling is usually a reliable signal of the severity of a fracture or dislocation.

    T—[F]

11. Which of the following are common signals of a fracture or dislocation?

   I. Deformity
   II. Inability to move an extremity
   III. Bruising of the skin
   IV. Pulselessness in an extremity
   V. Swelling over the site

   a. I and IV
   b. II and V
   c. I, II, III, and V
   d. All of the above

Objective 3

12. Pain, swelling, and any deformity are generally confined to the joint area in most sprains.

   [T]—F

13. You should suspect a serious musculoskeletal injury if the victim tells you that she—

   a. Has a slight pain in her ankle when she walks.
   b. Heard a snap or pop when she struck the ground.
   c. Has a history of frequent prior dislocations.
   d. Notices that her injured wrist feels warm to the touch.

14. You would suspect a fracture or dislocation if—

   a. The victim could move the injured area without pain.
   b. The area was slightly swollen.
   c. The victim heard a snap at the time of the injury.
   d. a and b

Objective 4

15. You suspect a victim has sustained multiple musculoskeletal injuries. You should call EMS personnel.

   [T]—F

Objective 5

16. Which of the following are included in your general care for musculoskeletal injuries?

   a. Ice and gentle exercise
   b. Rest, ice, and elevation
   c. Splints, bandaging, and elevation
   d. Rest and heat packs

17. You should immobilize a musculoskeletal injury in order to—

   a. Prevent further soft tissue damage.
   b. Lessen pain.
   c. Lessen the danger of infection.
   d. All of the above

18. Your care for both an open and a closed fracture may include an ice pack to help reduce swelling or pain.

   T—[F]

19. Applying ice and elevating the injured part first will make it easier to splint a musculoskeletal injury.

   T—[F]

20. You have splinted a suspected closed fracture of the forearm and determined that the victim has no other injuries. It would now be appropriate for you to transport the victim to a medical facility.

   [T]—F

Objective 6

21. What must you do to effectively immobilize a fracture of the forearm?

   a. Include the wrist and forearm in the splint.
   b. Include the fingers, hand, wrist, and forearm in the splint.
   c. Include the forearm and elbow in the splint.
   d. Include the wrist, forearm, and elbow in the splint.

22. An effective splint should do all of the following **except—**

   a. Prevent a closed fracture from becoming an open fracture.
   b. Decrease circulation to the injured area and minimize swelling.
   c. Lessen pain and increase the victim's comfort.
   d. Reduce the risk of serious internal bleeding.

23. After you splint an extremity, the victim's toes or fingers below the splint should be a normal color but feel slightly cool to the touch.

T—[F]

24. Which would you do to correctly splint a suspected fracture of the lower leg?

    a. Apply a rigid splint padded to fit the deformity and secure with cravats.

    b. Leave the leg unsplinted until the victim can be moved to an ambulance.

    c. Have a bystander help you straighten the leg before you apply a rigid splint.

    d. Bandage the leg using bulky dressings to immobilize the fracture area.

25. The three types of splints available to the citizen responder are soft, rigid, and—

    a. Commercial.

    b. Improvised.

    c. Anatomic.

    d. Traction.

26. Tying a victim's fractured leg to the other leg does not effectively splint the fracture.

T—[F]

Objective 7

27. Match each term on the right with the definition on the left. Put its letter on the line in front of the definition.

Answer	Definition		Term
c	A gradual, progressive weakening of bone	a.	Dislocation
d	The stretching and tearing of ligaments and other soft tissues at a joint	b.	Fracture
a	The displacement of a bone from its normal position at a joint	c.	Osteoporosis
e	The stretching and tearing of muscles and tendons	d.	Sprain
b	A break or disruption in bone tissue	e.	Strain

Chapter 10—Injuries to the Head and Spine

Objective 1

1. The most common cause of head and spine injuries is diving into shallow water.

T—[F]

2. Nearly half of all head and spine injuries are the result of—

    a. Sports mishaps.

    b. Motor vehicle crashes.

    c. Falls from heights.

    d. Assaults and attacks.

Objective 2

3. For which of the following people should you consider the possibility of a serious head and/or spine injury?

    a. An 18-year-old who fell from a height of 3 feet

    b. A helmeted motorcyclist whose helmet was cracked as he hit the ground

    c. A conscious victim of a motor vehicle crash who was not wearing a seat belt

    d. b and c

4. Because a person is found unconscious with no visible wounds or bleeding from the head, it is possible to rule out a serious head injury.

T—[F]

5. A person has a gunshot wound in the abdomen. You should care for him or her as a possible spinal injury victim.

[T]—F

Objective 3

6. Which is often the first and most important signal of a serious head injury?

    a. Blood or fluid in the ears

    b. Altered level of consciousness

    c. Severe pain or pressure in the head

    d. Seizures or convulsions

7. Which of the following is **not** a signal of head or spine injury?

   a. Tingling in the extremities
   b. Partial or complete paralysis
   c. Confusion about the hour or day
   d. Elevated body temperature

8. Nausea or vomiting is one of the signals of head and/or spine injuries.

   [T]—F

Objective 4

9. Which is the most important step in your care of a spinal injury victim?

   a. Minimize movement of the head and spine.
   b. Maintain an open airway.
   c. Monitor level of consciousness.
   d. Maintain normal body temperature.

10. You should maintain in-line stabilization of a victim with possible spinal injury until—

    a. The head is in line with the body.
    b. The victim indicates that head and neck pain is reduced.
    c. Care of the victim is assumed by EMS personnel.
    d. The victim's airway is clear and breathing is eased.

11. You should expect to feel some resistance when bringing the head of a spinal injury victim in line with the body. You should continue gentle movement until the head has been brought to the anatomically normal position.

    T—[F]

Objective 5

12. You wish to control bleeding from a scalp wound. The skull appears uninjured. You should apply firm direct pressure over the wound with a clean dressing.

    [T]—F

13. From which part of the body should you remove an impaled object if necessary to control bleeding?

    a. Chest
    b. Cheek
    c. Eye
    d. Hand

14. In most cases, the proper position for a victim of a nosebleed is sitting with head tilted back.

    T—[F]

15. A piece of glass has become impaled in a victim's eye. Assuming the victim has no other injuries or problems, which would you do first?

    a. Place a sterile dressing around the object and control bleeding surrounding the eye.
    b. Stabilize the object with bulky dressings and a paper cup to secure it in place.
    c. Place the victim on the back.
    d. Cover the uninjured eye to prevent blinking or other eye movement which might increase eye damage.

16. You should never remove a foreign object you can see in a victim's ear canal.

    T—[F]

17. Which is the proper first aid care for an injured person showing blood or fluid discharge from the right ear?

    a. Place the victim on the right side with the involved ear down.
    b. Cover the ear lightly with a sterile dressing.
    c. Control the discharge with direct pressure and gauze packing.
    d. Leave the ear uncovered to drain, and elevate the head.

18. A victim has sustained a blow that caused a wound inside the mouth. You do not suspect head or spine injury. Which is the preferred position for this victim?

    a. Sitting with her head tilted slightly forward
    b. Sitting with her head tilted slightly back
    c. Lying on her back with head tilted to the side
    d. Lying on her side

19. A knocked-out tooth should be preserved in alcohol and transported with the victim for possible replantation.

    T—[F]

20. You may need to apply pressure to both carotid arteries to control severe bleeding in the neck.

    T—[F]

Objective 6

21. Which of the following actions can help to prevent head and spine injuries?

    I. Safeguarding your home against falls
    II. Teaching your children about bike safety
    III. Eating a balanced diet and exercising regularly
    IV. Following the rules in sports activities
    V. Avoiding exercising in extreme heat

    ---

    a. I, II, IV, and V
    b. I, II, and IV
    c. III and V
    d. All of the above

Objective 7

22. Match each term on the right with its definition on the left. Puts its letter on the line in front of the definition.

e	The 33 bones that form the spine	a.	Concussion
d	A bundle of nerves extending from the base of the skull to the lower back	b.	In-line stabilization
a	A temporary impairment of brain function, usually without permanent damage to the brain	c.	Intervertebral
b	A technique to minimize movement of a victim's head and neck	d.	Spinal cord
		e.	Vertebrae

Chapter 11—Injuries to the Chest, Abdomen, and Pelvis

Objective 1

1. An injury to the abdomen from a blunt object may result in fatal bleeding because of injury to the—

    a. Liver.
    b. Spleen.
    c. Stomach.
    d. All of the above

2. A victim of an automobile crash has suffered injury to the chest. She may also have a spinal injury.

    [T]—F

3. Fracture of the pelvis can result in injury to the bladder, rectum, and kidneys.

    T—[F]

Objective 2

4. Which should be included in your basic care for serious chest or abdominal injuries?

    I. Calling EMS personnel
    II. Administering oxygen
    III. Applying ice or cold packs
    IV. Minimizing shock
    V. Limiting victim movement

    ---

    a. I, II, and IV
    b. II and V
    c. I, III, IV, and V
    d. I, IV, and V

5. Victims of serious chest or abdominal injuries may develop the signals of shock resulting from—

    a. Loss of blood into the chest or abdomen.
    b. Breathing difficulty.
    c. Severe pain from fractures and wounds.
    d. All of the above

Objective 3

6. Which signal might indicate a serious chest injury?

    a. Unusually warm skin around the ribs
    b. Coughing up blood
    c. Slow, deep inhalations and exhalations
    d. A series of respirations increasing in rate and depth followed by a pause

7. A victim who is having difficulty breathing because of a serious chest injury may have a flushed or bluish discoloration of the skin.

    [T]—F

Objective 4

8. Which position will a victim of a simple rib fracture often take?

   a. Lying flat on the back
   b. Lying flat on the stomach
   c. Sitting with the shoulders back and chest out
   d. Sitting with a hand or arm supporting the chest

9. A victim with a suspected simple rib fracture does not need to be seen or transported by EMS personnel.

   T—[F]

Objective 5

10. What is the primary signal of a sucking chest wound?

    a. Increasing shortness of breath and coughing
    b. A crackly sensation under the skin when the chest is touched
    c. The sound of air passing in and out of the wound during breathing
    d. A portion of the chest moving opposite to the rest during breathing

11. The most important first aid care for a sucking chest wound is to control the bleeding that occurs around the opening in the chest.

    T—[F]

12. What dressing should be used first to care for a sucking chest wound?

    a. Gauze pads
    b. Universal dressing
    c. Adhesive compress
    d. Airtight dressing

Objective 6

13. When caring for a victim with serious abdominal injuries, which threat to life is your primary concern?

    a. Bleeding
    b. Infection
    c. Respiratory distress
    d. Diabetic coma

14. Which signals indicate possible serious abdominal injury?

    I. Nausea and vomiting
    II. Respiratory distress
    III. Weakness and thirst
    IV. Coughing blood
    V. Bruising

    ---

    a. I and II
    b. III and IV
    c. I, III, and V
    d. II and III

Objective 7

15. In which position should you place the victim of a closed abdominal injury?

    a. Lying flat on the back with the legs raised about 12 inches
    b. Lying on the back with the knees flexed and supported by a blanket
    c. Lying on the side with legs drawn up toward the abdomen
    d. Semisitting with knees flexed and supported by a blanket

16. A bullet has entered the front of a victim's abdomen and you find no exit wound. What appears to be part of the intestine is protruding from the wound. How would you care for this wound?

    a. Put moist sterile dressings loosely over the wound.
    b. Apply direct pressure on a sterile dressing over the wound.
    c. Cover the wound with dry gauze pads and wrap roller gauze around the body.
    d. Leave the area uncovered to prevent contaminating the intestine.

17. To protect a protruding intestine, you would cover the intestine with a dry sterile dressing, cover the dressing loosely with plastic wrap, and apply heat.

    T—[F]

Objective 6

18. Which of the following might indicate a pelvic injury?
    a. Shortening of one leg
    b. Outward rotation of the left foot
    c. Loss of sensation in the legs
    d. All of the above

Objective 7

19. Which of the following is part of the first aid care for a victim of a suspected pelvic fracture?
    a. Rolling the victim to a position lying flat on the back
    b. Placing the victim on one side with the knees flexed toward the abdomen
    c. Moving the victim to a semisitting position unless pain is increased
    d. Not moving the victim from the position found unless necessary

Objective 8

20. Since a victim who has sustained an injury to the genitals may become embarrassed as you attempt to apply a dressing to the area, you should explain briefly what you are going to do and then proceed without hesitation.

    [T]—F

Objective 9

21. The long, flat bone in the middle of the front of the rib cage is the—
    a. Sternum.
    b. Femur.
    c. Clavicle.
    d. Scapula.

Chapter 12—Injuries to the Extremities

Objective 1

1. A child has fallen from a skateboard and landed on an elbow. What signals would you expect to see if the elbow is seriously injured?
    I. Pain in the wrist
    II. Deformity at the elbow
    III. Swelling and discoloration of the elbow
    IV. Paralysis of the hand

    ---

    a. All of the above
    b. I and IV
    c. II and III
    d. I, II, and III

Objective 2

2. Suspected fractures or dislocations of the arm can be effectively immobilized by binding the injured arm to the victim's chest.

    [T]—F

3. In which position does a victim of a clavicle fracture usually sit or stand?
    a. Shoulders pulled back and both arms at the sides
    b. Holding the arm on the injured side against the chest
    c. Uninjured side bent forward and that arm against the chest
    d. Arm on the injured side dangling loosely at the side of the body

4. The most common signal of a fractured scapula is deformity at the point of fracture.

    T—[F]

5. Which is a frequent cause of shoulder dislocations?
    a. Movement of the arm outside the normal range of motion
    b. A heavy blow to the front or back of the shoulder area
    c. Violent pulling action on the arm, forearm, or hand
    d. Falling on an outstretched arm

6. How should you immobilize a serious shoulder injury?

   a. Allow the victim to continue to support the arm and immobilize it in that position.

   b. Gently straighten the arm, apply a rigid splint, and secure it to the victim's body.

   c. Use pillows, blankets, or other padding to fill any gaps between the arm and the victim's body.

   d. a and c

7. Which structures must you immobilize to effectively care for a suspected fracture of the upper arm?

   a. Humerus and elbow

   b. Humerus, elbow, and forearm

   c. Shoulder, humerus, and elbow

   d. Shoulder, humerus, elbow, and forearm

8. Placing the injured arm in a sling and binding it to the chest with cravats is an effective technique for splinting a fracture of the upper arm.

   [T]—F

9. In which position should you immobilize a suspected fracture or dislocation of the elbow?

   a. Slightly flexed with a rigid splint spanning and secured to the elbow

   b. Straight, immobilized with a rigid splint, and secured against the trunk

   c. Forearm supported in a sling and the upper arm secured to the body

   d. Any of the above, maintaining the position in which the elbow is found

Objective 3

10. Fractures of the forearm are more common in adults than in children.

    T—[F]

11. Since finger dislocations can often be easily and safely brought back into place with a quick in-line pull, a single attempt to do so is an acceptable part of your first aid care for this injury.

    T—[F]

12. Which of the following should be included in the immobilization of a suspected forearm fracture?

    I. A rigid splint secured from the site of the injury to the hand

    II. A roll of gauze or dressing material to keep the hand in a normal position

    III. A sling to support the forearm across the chest

    IV. Cravats to secure the arm to the victim's chest

    a. I and II

    b. I, III, and IV

    c. II, III, and IV

    d. IV

Objective 4

13. Which of the following signals would you expect to see if a victim has fractured the left femur?

    a. The left leg shortened and foot turned inward

    b. The left leg lengthened and foot turned inward

    c. The left leg shortened and foot turned outward

    d. The left leg lengthened and foot turned outward

Objective 5

14. You have splinted a victim's suspected closed fracture of the lower leg. He has no other injuries. It may be appropriate to transport him to the hospital yourself rather than calling EMS personnel.

    T—[F]

15. You find a victim with a fractured femur lying with the injured thigh against the ground. You should not move it since the ground will provide an effective splint.

    [T]—F

16. You are providing first aid to a man who was struck by a car on the side of his right knee. A laceration on the front of the knee is bleeding moderately. He cannot move the knee without pain. Which of the following should you include as your first aid care?

   I. Elevate the leg.
   II. Control the bleeding.
   III. Support the knee in the position you found it.
   IV. Straighten the leg and secure to the uninjured leg.
   V. Transport the victim to the hospital yourself if he requests it.

   ---

   a. I, II, III, and IV
   b. III and V
   c. II and III
   d. III and V

Objective 6

17. Which signals indicate that an injury to the foot or ankle needs to be evaluated by a physician?
   a. The ankle or foot is painful to move.
   b. The victim cannot bear weight on the ankle or foot.
   c. The foot or ankle is swollen.
   d. All of the above

18. Which should you use to splint an injured ankle and foot?
   a. A rigid splint from the lower leg to the foot
   b. A rigid splint along the back of the leg extending beyond the knee and ankle
   c. An elastic bandage covering from six inches above the ankle to the toes
   d. A pillow wrapped around the foot and ankle and secured with three cravats

Objective 7

19. Match each term on the right with its definition on the left. Put its letter on the line in front of the definition.

g	Shoulder blade	a.	Clavicle
a	Collarbone	b.	Femur
d	Upper arm	c.	Fibula
b	Thighbone	d.	Humerus
e	Kneecap	e.	Patella
		f.	Radius
		g.	Scapula

Chapter 13—Medical Emergencies (Introduction) and Sudden Illnesses

Objective 2

1. Which of the following is **not** one of the basics of first aid care for medical emergencies?
   a. Do no further harm.
   b. Monitor the ABCs.
   c. Notify EMS personnel.
   d. Get a medical history.

Objective 1

2. Which of the following are considered general signals of sudden illness?
   a. Change in level of consciousness
   b. Slowing pulse and breathing rates
   c. Nausea and vomiting
   d. All of the above

3. To safely choose the right first aid care for a victim of a sudden illness, you must have a clear idea of what is causing the signals you see in the victim.

   T—[F]

Objective 2

4. Which is the primary cause of fainting?

   a. A temporary spasm of the arteries in the brain

   b. A rupture of a small blood vessel in the brain

   c. A temporary reduction of blood flow to the brain

   d. A sudden increase in the volume of blood in the brain

5. A person about to faint will frequently resemble a person going into shock.

   [T]—F

6. Your first aid care for a victim of fainting should include—

   I. Placing the victim in a semisitting position.

   II. Elevating the victim's legs.

   III. Giving a conscious victim small sips of water or fruit juice.

   IV. Conducting a primary survey.

   V. Splashing water on the victim's face.

   a. I, III, and V

   b. II, IV, and V

   c. I and III

   d. II and IV

Objective 3

7. Diabetes mellitus is a condition in which the body produces more insulin than is needed to process the sugar that the person is eating.

   T—[F]

8. Since improper treatment of a diabetic emergency can be fatal to the victim, you must distinguish between hyperglycemia and hypoglycemia before providing first aid to a diabetic who has suddenly become ill.

   T—[F]

9. Which signals would you see in a victim of a diabetic emergency?

   a. Rapid pulse, slow breathing, changes in consciousness

   b. Rapid pulse, rapid breathing, changes in consciousness

   c. Normal pulse, rapid breathing, normal consciousness

   d. Slow pulse, normal breathing, normal consciousness

10. Which should you include in your care for a conscious person who exhibits the signals of a diabetic emergency?

    a. Helping him or her to administer insulin

    b. Giving sugar water or fruit juice to drink

    c. Doing a secondary survey

    d. b and c

11. If you closely monitor and maintain the airway, it is acceptable to place a small amount of dry sugar or honey under the tongue of an unconscious diabetic.

    T—[F]

12. A friend who is a diabetic is drowsy and seems confused. He is not sure if he took his insulin that day. What should you do?

    a. Give him some sugar.

    b. Suggest he rest for an hour or so.

    c. Tell him to take his insulin.

    d. b and c

Objective 4

13. In caring for a victim having a seizure, you should—

    a. Move any objects that might cause injury.

    b. Try to hold the person still.

    c. Place a spoon between the person's teeth.

    d. Douse the person with water.

14. Which type of sudden illness may be preceded by an aura?

    a. Fainting

    b. Diabetic coma

    c. Seizure

    d. Heart attack

15. A woman in your office falls to the floor and begins to exhibit violent, uncontrolled movement. Which of the following first aid steps should you take?

    I. Hold the woman to protect her from injury.

    II. Place a pillow or thick folded blanket under her head to protect it.

    III. Place a pencil, ruler, or similar object between her teeth, if possible.

    IV. Place the victim on her side when the seizure subsides.

    V. Do a secondary survey following the seizure.

    ---

    a. I, II, and IV

    b. II, III, and V

    c. IV and V

    d. All of the above

Objective 5

16. In which circumstance should you call EMS personnel to provide care for a victim of a seizure?

    a. The victim is pregnant.

    b. The victim is a child.

    c. The victim has no history of seizures.

    d. All of the above

17. You do not need to call EMS personnel to see a victim who recovers from a seizure within a few minutes, is not injured, and tells you that he has never had a seizure before.

    T—[F]

Objective 6

18. Two risk factors of stroke that you can control are lack of exercise and cigarette smoking.

    [T]—F

19. How much greater is the risk of having a stroke for a person with uncontrolled hypertension than for a person with normal blood pressure?

    a. Twice the risk

    b. Three times the risk

    c. Five times the risk

    d. Seven times the risk

Objective 7

20. Which signals would make you suspect that a person has had a stroke?

    I. Numbness and tingling in both arms

    II. Pupils of unequal size

    III. Intense ringing in the ears

    IV. Slurred speech

    V. Loss of bladder control

    ---

    a. I, II, and IV

    b. II, III, IV, and V

    c. I and V

    d. All of the above

21. Which is the best position in which to place a stroke victim who is drooling or having difficulty swallowing?

    a. Semisitting, head raised

    b. Lying on one side

    c. Lying flat on the back

    d. Lying on the back, legs elevated

22. The most immediate first aid step you should take with an unconscious victim is to—

    a. Call EMS personnel.

    b. Comfort and reassure the victim.

    c. Open the airway and check breathing.

    d. Move the victim to a position on one side.

Objective 8

23. Match each term on the right with its definition on the left. Put its letter on the line in front of the definition.

    __h__ Temporary disruption of blood flow to the brain

    __b__ An unusual sensation or feeling preceding a seizure

    __c__ Condition in which the body does not produce enough insulin

    __e__ A condition in which too much sugar is in the blood

    __a__ A weak area in an artery wall

    a. Aneurysm

    b. Aura

    c. Diabetes mellitus

    d. Epilepsy

    e. Hyper-glycemia

    f. Hypo-glycemia

    g. Stroke

    h. TIA

Chapter 14—Poisoning, Bites, and Stings

Objective 1

1. Which types of substances are responsible for the largest percentage of unintentional poisonings?

   a. Cleaning products
   b. Foods
   c. Petroleum products
   d. Drugs and medications

2. The four ways poisons enter the body are ingestion, injection, inhalation, and insufflation.

   T—[F]

Objective 2

3. When approaching a person who may be the victim of poisoning, which should be the first step you take?

   a. Surveying the scene
   b. Interviewing the bystanders
   c. Doing a primary survey
   d. Doing a secondary survey

4. Which signal would help you differentiate a victim of poisoning from a victim of another medical emergency?

   a. Nausea, vomiting, and abdominal pain
   b. Breathing difficulty
   c. Burns around the lips and tongue
   d. Seizures and loss of consciousness

5. Which of the following questions should you ask about a suspected poisoning to assist you in providing first aid?

   I. Who was with the victim before the poisoning took place?
   II. What type of poison was taken?
   III. How much was taken?
   IV. Does the victim have a history of drug abuse?
   V. When was the poison taken?
   VI. Has the victim been depressed or threatening suicide?

   ---

   a. All of the above
   b. I, II, IV, and VI
   c. I and V
   d. II, III, and V

6. You suspect a poisoning. You should try to discover whether the victim has a history of drug misuse or abuse. This information is needed to help you decide the specific care you will provide.

   T—[F]

Objective 3

7. You suspect that a conscious victim has been exposed to a poison. Your first call should be to—

   a. 9–1–1 or a local emergency number.
   b. The person's physician.
   c. The Poison Control Center.
   d. The hospital emergency department.

8. You suspect that a victim is unconscious as a result of a poisoning. Your first call should be to—

   a. 9–1–1 or a local emergency number.
   b. The hospital emergency department.
   c. The Poison Control Center.
   d. The Drug Information Center.

Objective 4

9. Which is your first responsibility in assisting a victim of poisoning?

   a. Assessing the victim's ABCs
   b. Calling the Poison Control Center
   c. Safeguarding yourself and the victim from further exposure to the poison
   d. Gathering items that will help EMS personnel identify the poison

10. A person who has ingested a poison is conscious. You should give him water to drink as soon as possible to dilute the poison. Then you should call the Poison Control Center for further instructions.

    T—[F]

Objective 5

11. Which is the normal dose of syrup of ipecac for a child under the age of 12?

    a. One teaspoon
    b. One tablespoon
    c. Two tablespoons
    d. Three tablespoons

12. In which of the following ingested poisoning situations might the Poison Control Center tell you to induce a victim to vomit?

    a. **Less than 30 minutes has passed since the poisoning.**
    b. More than three hours has passed since the poisoning.
    c. The poison is a petroleum product.
    d. The victim is unconscious.

13. Which of the following poisons should not be eliminated by inducing vomiting?

    a. Poisonous berries
    b. **Corrosive cleansers, such as drain cleaner**
    c. Sleeping pills
    d. Aspirin

14. Which of the following might be used in the first aid care for a poisoning victim?

    a. Activated charcoal
    b. Paregoric
    c. Syrup of ipecac
    d. **a and c**

15. The correct dose of activated charcoal for a person age 1 to 12 years is four tablespoons in a glass of water.

    [T]—F

16. For which of the following ingested poisons might you be told to give a conscious victim water to dilute the poison?

    a. **Corrosive chemicals**
    b. Drug tablets or capsules
    c. Petroleum products
    d. All of the above

17. Which signal are you likely to see in a victim in the early stages of carbon monoxide poisoning?

    a. **Pale or bluish skin color**
    b. Cherry-red skin color
    c. Profuse sweating
    d. Hot, dry, red skin

18. You come across a victim who has inhaled a poison. Your first step in assisting the victim is to—

    a. Provide supplemental oxygen.
    b. Administer rescue breathing.
    c. **Get him or her away from the poisonous substance and call EMS personnel.**
    d. Do a primary survey to determine if he or she is breathing.

19. If you are exposed to poison ivy or poison oak, you should—

    a. Wash the affected area with hydrogen peroxide.
    b. Wash the affected area with soap and water.
    c. Apply a baking soda paste to any rash or lesions.
    d. **b and c**

20. In cases of exposure to a dry chemical such as lime, you should brush all visible particles from the affected area before flushing the area with running water.

    T—[F]

Objective 6

21. How should you remove a stinger embedded in a victim's skin?

    a. Use a tweezers to pull it out.
    b. **Scrape it away from the skin with a fingernail or plastic card.**
    c. Use a small sewing needle to pull it from the skin.
    d. Any of the above techniques is acceptable.

22. Applying warm moist packs to insect stings will help reduce pain and swelling.

    T—[F]

23. How can you identify a brown recluse spider?

    a. By the brown color of its body
    b. By the hourglass shape on its underbody
    c. **By the dark brown violin-shaped marking on the top of its body**
    d. By the thick brown hairs on its legs

24. Signals of certain spider bites and scorpion stings include profuse sweating and salivating, irregular heart rhythms, and severe pain and swelling in the sting or bite area.

    [T]—F

25. Which should you do for the victim of a scorpion sting while waiting for EMS personnel?

    a. Wash the wound and apply a cold pack.

    b. Wash the wound and apply a hot pack.

    c. Keep the wound area dry and elevate the involved extremity.

    d. Keep the involved extremity lower than the heart and apply a sterile dressing.

26. For which sting would application of meat tenderizer be an appropriate first aid technique?

    a. Scorpion sting

    b. Wasp sting

    c. Jellyfish sting

    d. Honeybee sting

27. In which situations involving a marine animal sting should you call EMS personnel?

    a. The specific cause of the sting is unknown.

    b. The victim has a history of allergic reactions to stings.

    c. The sting occurred on the face.

    d. All of the above.

28. In providing first aid to a victim of a snakebite, you should **not**—

    a. Clean the wound with soap and water.

    b. Splint the affected part.

    c. Keep the affected part lower than the heart.

    d. Apply ice or a cold pack to the area of the bite.

29. You should suction a snakebite only if the victim cannot get to medical care within—

    a. 30 minutes.

    b. 20 minutes.

    c. 15 minutes.

    d. 10 minutes.

30. You should apply an ice or cold pack to the site of a snakebite as soon as possible to slow the absorption of the venom.

    T—[F]

31. You can effectively remove a tick from the skin by touching the tick with a hot match or coating it with petroleum jelly.

    T—[F]

32. The best way to remove a tick from the skin is to—

    a. Coat the tick with nail polish.

    b. Burn the tick with a hot match.

    c. Grasp the tick close to the skin and pull slowly.

    d. Scrape the tick from the skin with a fingernail or credit card.

33. The typical first sign of an infection resulting from the bite of a tick carrying Lyme disease consists of—

    a. Small blisters.

    b. A red, raised rash.

    c. Numerous red, swollen areas.

    d. Dry flaky patches.

34. Once a tick has been removed from the skin, you should immediately wash the area of the bite with soap and water and coat it with an antiseptic or antibiotic ointment.

    [T]—F

35. The first signal in most cases of Lyme disease is a red, raised rash. The rash often looks like a bull's-eye around the site of the bite.

    [T]—F

36. In caring for an insect sting, you should—

    a. Remove remaining stinger by scraping it from the skin.

    b. Remove remaining stinger using tweezers.

    c. Wash the sting site, then cover it.

    d. a and c

Objective *7*

37. When spending time outdoors in woods or tall grass, to prevent bites and stings you should—

    a. Wear dark-colored clothing.

    b. Wear loose-fitting clothing.

    c. Tuck pant legs into boots or socks.

    d. All of the above

38. Which will help protect you from insect and tick bites?

I. Wearing long-sleeved shirts and long pants in wooded areas

II. Walking or hiking early in the morning or around dusk

III. Taping the area where your pants and socks meet

IV. Wearing dark clothes, which are less attractive to insects and ticks

V. Spraying repellent on pets that go outdoors

a. All of the above

b. II, IV, and V

c. I, III, and V

d. I, II, and III

Objective 6

39. In general, the first aid care for an animal bite is the same as for any other wound.

[T]—F

40. Which is included in the proper first aid for an animal bite?

a. Washing the wound with soap and water

b. Restraining or capturing the animal

c. Calling the humane society

d. All of the above

Objective 7

41. An insect and tick repellent containing permethrin is considered safe for use on both skin and clothing.

T—[F]

Objective 9

42. Anaphylaxis develops slowly and is often overshadowed by more obvious medical problems in a first aid situation.

T—[F]

43. Which signals are you likely to see in a victim of anaphylaxis?

a. Hives, rash, itching

b. Nausea, vomiting

c. Coughing, wheezing

d. All of the above

44. Which body system is most likely to be the focus of life-threatening problems in anaphylaxis?

a. Integumentary

b. Musculoskeletal

c. Circulatory

d. Respiratory

Objective 10

45. The majority of child poisoning cases occur while the child is under the direct supervision of a parent or guardian.

[T]—F

Objective 11

46. Match each term on the right with its definition on the left. Put its letter on the line in front of the definition.

e	A substance that causes injury, illness, or death when introduced into the body.	a.	Activated charcoal
f	A substance used to induce vomiting in poisoning cases	b.	Antivenin
a	A substance used to absorb ingested poisons	c.	Baking soda
b	A substance used in the treatment of poisoning from the bites of certain snakes and spiders.	d.	Epinephrine
d	A chemical used in insect and tick repellants	e.	DEET
		f.	Poison
		g.	Syrup of ipecac

Chapter 15—Substance Misuse and Abuse

Objective 1

1. Which are the major categories of commonly abused or misused substances?

a. Medications, alcohol, and cocaine

b. Stimulants, hallucinogens, and depressants

c. Inhalants, amphetamines, and narcotics

d. Alcohol, cocaine, and heroin

2. A smokable form of methamphetamine that has extremely addictive properties is called—

   a. Crack.
   b. Angel dust.
   c. Mesc.
   d. Ice.

3. Caffeine and nicotine are both categorized as stimulants.

   [T]—F

4. Which signals are you likely to observe in a person who has taken an overdose of amphetamines?

   a. Slurred speech, drowsiness, confusion, nausea
   b. Profound depression, slow pulse, dilated pupils, thirst
   c. Sweating, chills, rapid pulse, restlessness
   d. Euphoria, dry skin, flushed face, increased appetite

5. Mescaline, phencyclidine, and psilocybin are drugs categorized as—

   a. Stimulants.
   b. Depressants.
   c. Hallucinogens.
   d. Narcotics.

6. The physical effects you would notice in a person who has ingested a hallucinogenic drug would be similar to those produced by a depressant.

   T—[F]

7. Narcotics, alcohol, and barbiturates are substances categorized as—

   a. Stimulants.
   b. Depressants.
   c. Hallucinogens.
   d. Narcotics.

8. Chronic use of anabolic steroids can cause serious side effects, including—

   a. Lung cancer and strokes.
   b. Kidney failure and ulcers.
   c. Sterility and liver cancer.
   d. Hypertension and arthritis.

9. Misuse of aspirin may cause temporary discomfort but is unlikely to do any long-term damage to the victim.

   T—[F]

Objective 2

10. Which of the following is true of substance abuse?

    a. It occurs only among those elderly who are forgetful and/or may have poor eyesight.
    b. It is the use of a substance for intended purposes but in improper amounts or doses.
    c. It is the use of a substance without regard to health concerns or accepted medical practices.
    d. Its effects are minor and rarely result in medical complications.

11. Using leftover prescription medication that is outdated will probably do no harm.

    T—[F]

12. To avoid an unintentional misuse or overdose of a prescription drug, you should know the—

    a. Effects of the drug.
    b. Potential side effects of the drug.
    c. Drugs with which it will interact.
    d. All of the above

Objective 3

13. You are walking home from a movie and notice a man in front of you stumble and fall. He gets to his feet and walks unsteadily toward you. You ask him if he's all right, and he replies incoherently. He stumbles again and falls. You notice a smell of alcohol on his breath. Which of the conditions below could cause this person's problems?

    a. Depressant overdose
    b. Alcohol intoxication
    c. Hyperglycemia
    d. All of the above

14. Which signals are you likely to observe in a person who has taken an overdose of depressants?

    a. Slurred speech, drowsiness, confusion
    b. Paranoia, rapid pulse, pinpoint pupils
    c. Sweating, chills, rapid pulse
    d. Euphoria, dry skin, flushed face

15. Hallucinations are a signal occurring both with ingestion of drugs such as LSD and in withdrawal from alcohol.

[T]—F

Objective 4

16. The first aid care for emergencies arising from substance abuse follows the same general principles as those for poisoning.

[T]—F

Objective 5

17. Match each term on the right with its definition on the left. Put its letter on the line in front of the definition.

a	Compulsive need to use a substance to prevent withdrawal	a.	Addiction
d	Substances that alter perceptions of time and space and produce delusions	b.	Dependency
h	Condition occurring when a substance user has to increase the dose and frequency of use of the substance to obtain the desired effect	c.	Depressants
g	The use of a substance for an unintended purpose	d.	Hallucinogens
e	Substances that affect the central nervous system to speed up mental and physical activity	e.	Stimulants
		f.	Substance abuse
		g.	Substance misuse
		h.	Tolerance

Chapter 16—Heat and Cold Emergencies

Objective 1

1. Which major mechanisms does the body use to remove heat?
   a. Constriction of blood vessels near the skin and shivering
   b. Dilation of the blood vessels near the skin and evaporation of sweat
   c. Reduction of body metabolism rate and increased breathing rate
   d. Increased metabolism of fat and reduced metabolism of carbohydrates

2. When the humidity in the environment is high, which of the body's mechanisms for removing excess heat is less effective?
   a. Dilation of surface blood vessels
   b. Increased breathing rate
   c. Evaporation of sweat
   d. Shivering

3. Shivering is one of the body's mechanisms for producing heat. It is used when constriction of the blood vessels near the skin cannot effectively maintain body temperature.

   [T]—F

4. Young children have a greater resistance to extremes of heat and cold than do middle-aged adults.

   T—[F]

5. A person who has had a heat- or cold-related illness in the past builds an immunity to the condition. He or she is less likely to fall victim to that illness again.

   T—[F]

6. You are giving first aid to a person who appears to be a victim of heat-related illness. Which type of medications could he be taking that would make him especially susceptible to heat- or cold-related illness?
   a. Stimulants
   b. Depressants
   c. Diuretics
   d. Analgesics

7. The three conditions that can result from overexposure to heat are—
   a. Heat cramps, heat shock, and heat strain.
   b. Heat stress, heat exhaustion, and heat strain.
   c. Heat sensitivity, heat shock, and heat stroke.
   d. Heat cramps, heat exhaustion, and heat stroke.

Objective 2

8. Heat cramps are usually associated with—
   a. Elevated body temperature.
   b. Heavy exercise outdoors.
   c. Dry, flushed skin.
   d. All of the above.

9. The signals of heat exhaustion are similar to those of—
   a. Diabetic emergency.
   b. Stroke.
   c. Shock.
   d. Narcotics overdose.

10. A victim of heat exhaustion will frequently have dry, pale skin, elevated body temperature, and a rapid pulse.

    T—[F]

11. In heat stroke, the victim's body loses the ability to remove heat and its temperature rises to dangerous levels.

    [T]—F

12. A soccer player has collapsed at a game. The air temperature is 92°F and the humidity is high. You note that his skin is flushed and wet. He is breathing rapidly, has a weak pulse, and his face feels cool. What illness do you suspect?
    a. Stimulant overdose
    b. Heat-related illness
    c. Stroke
    d. Heart attack

13. Change in the victim's level of consciousness is one of the signals that the condition of the victim of a heat-related illness is worsening.

    [T]—F

Objective 3

14. As you are providing first aid to a victim of heat-related illness, which signals indicate that you should immediately call EMS personnel?
    a. The victim refuses water or vomits.
    b. The victim loses consciousness.
    c. The victim begins to sweat profusely.
    d. a and b

Objective 4

15. Which of the following steps is **not** part of the first aid care for a victim of heat cramps?
    a. Have the victim rest in a cool place.
    b. Lightly stretch and massage the area.
    c. Have the victim take salt tablets.
    d. Provide plain water or a sports drink.

16. Having a victim of heat cramps take salt tablets raises his or her risk of developing heat exhaustion or heat stroke.

    [T]—F

17. Which of the following should you do for a victim in the early stage of a heat-related illness?
    a. Move the victim to a cool place to rest.
    b. Give the victim cool water to drink.
    c. Watch the victim carefully for signs of a worsening condition.
    d. All of the above

18. How much water should you give a conscious victim of a heat-related illness?
    a. A glass (8 ounces) every 15 minutes
    b. One-half glass (4 ounces) every 15 minutes
    c. A glass (8 ounces) every hour
    d. As much as the victim will drink

19. If the victim of a suspected heat-related illness begins to lose consciousness, you should—
    a. Cool the body using wet sheets, towels, or cold packs.
    b. Cool the body by applying rubbing alcohol.
    c. Give cool water to drink.
    d. a and c

Objective 5

20. A person has been exposed to the cold. The skin on his feet has become yellow. He has no feeling in his feet. This individual is a victim of—

    a. Gangrene.

    b. Frostbite.

    c. Trench foot.

    d. Hypothermia.

Objective 6

21. You suspect a person is suffering from hypothermia. What do you expect to find when you check the pulse?

    a. Weak, rapid pulse

    b. Full, bounding pulse

    c. Slow, irregular pulse

    d. Normal rate and rhythm

22. A victim of hypothermia will usually show a glassy stare and an increasingly aggressive attitude as the condition worsens.

    T—[F]

23. Except in the case of immersion in water, a person will not develop hypothermia unless the air temperature is below freezing.

    T—[F]

24. People who have taken certain types of substances are at increased risk of developing hypothermia. These substances include—

    a. Alcohol and barbiturates.

    b. Amphetamines and hallucinogens.

    c. Aspirin and diuretics.

    d. Caffeine and nicotine.

Objective 7

25. Which should be your first step in providing first aid care to a victim of frostbite?

    a. Rub the frostbitten area gently with your hands.

    b. Immerse the frostbitten area in warm water.

    c. Cover the area with a clean, dry cloth or dressing.

    d. Determine whether the victim has been drinking alcohol.

26. Which would be the most appropriate water temperature in which to immerse a frostbitten foot?

    a. 105°–110° F

    b. 100°–105° F

    c. 90°–95° F

    d. 80°–85° F

27. When should you remove a frostbitten foot from the warm water in which you have immersed it?

    a. When feeling returns to the foot

    b. When the foot begins to become painful and begins to swell

    c. When the foot begins to turn red and feel warm

    d. When the toes begin to tingle and a pulse can be felt in the foot

Objective 8

28. Which first aid care should you provide for a victim of hypothermia?

    I. Remove any wet clothing and dry the victim.

    II. Immerse the victim in warm water, if possible.

    III. Give warm liquids to drink, if the victim is conscious.

    IV. Closely monitor the victim's condition.

    V. Handle the victim gently.

    ---

    a. I, II, and V

    b. II, III, and IV

    c. I, III, IV, and V

    d. All of the above

29. Immersing a hypothermia victim in warm water is a better method of first aid care than using hot water bottles, heating pads, or similar heat sources.

    T—[F]

30. Rough handling of a hypothermia victim may trigger disturbances in the victim's heart rhythm and lead to cardiac arrest.

    [T]—F

Objective 9

31. Precautions you can take that will help you prevent both heat- and cold-related illnesses include—
    a. Keeping a constant, measured pace of activity while outdoors.
    b. Always wearing appropriate clothing for the environment.
    c. Drinking plenty of fluids.
    d. b and c

32. A few cups of coffee provide caffeine, which helps the body maintain its normal temperature while working outdoors in a cold environment.

    T—[F]

Objective 10

33. Match each term on the right with its definition on the left. Put its letter on the line in front of the definition.

Answer	Definition		Term
c	A condition in which body tissues freeze	a.	Benzodiazepines
d	A form of shock resulting from strenuous physical efforts in hot environments	b.	Diuretics
b	Medications that eliminate water from the body	c.	Frostbite
g	A figure that represents the combination of the temperature and wind speed	d.	Heat exhaustion
f	A condition in which the body's warming mechanisms fail and the entire body cools	e.	Heat stroke
		f.	Hypothermia
		g.	Wind chill

Chapter 17—Reaching and Moving Victims

Objective 1

1. In which of the following situations would you move a victim before providing first aid care?
    a. A victim lying in a supermarket aisle where a large crowd has gathered, obstructing the aisle
    b. A victim sitting in his truck on the shoulder of a busy highway; the truck's engine is running
    c. A victim unconscious in his car in a closed garage; the car's engine is running
    d. A victim who has fallen on her back in the bleachers at a high school football game; it is raining.

2. You should move a victim before providing first aid care if there is immediate danger to the victim or responder.

    T—[F]

3. You find a victim lying on the shoulder of the road next to an overturned car. You should move the victim away from the car before providing first aid care.

    T—[F]

4. Your decision about whether or not to move a victim before providing first aid care should be made when you complete your secondary survey.

    T—[F]

Objective 2

5. Which of the following should you consider to assure that you move a victim quickly and safely?
    a. Whether bystanders are available to help
    b. The size of the victim
    c. The victim's condition
    d. All of the above

6. You are deciding whether or not to attempt to pull a victim away from a burning car. Which of the following will help you make the decision?
    a. The victim weighs about 80 pounds more than you.
    b. There are four bystanders willing to help.
    c. The area around the victim is damp with gas.
    d. All of the above

Objective 3

7. How can you protect yourself from injury when moving a victim?

   a. Lift with your legs and back.

   b. Walk slowly backward rather than forward.

   c. Bend your body at the knees and hips.

   d. Use as long strides as you can comfortably take.

8. How can you help protect a victim from further injury when moving him or her in an emergency?

   a. Move the victim in a sitting position whenever possible.

   b. Roll the victim rather than pulling him or her from the head or feet.

   c. Keep the victim's head and neck supported during the movement.

   d. All of the above

9. When moving a victim, you can increase your stability and decrease your risk of stumbling by taking longer strides.

   T—[F]

Objective 4

10. The fireman's carry should **not** be used for—

    a. A victim of a heart attack.

    b. A victim who is unconscious.

    c. A victim of an abdominal injury.

    d. b and c

11. The fireman's carry is most useful when moving a victim who is substantially heavier than the rescuer.

    T—[F]

12. To place a victim in the fireman's carry, you must—

    a. Support the victim who is standing next to you.

    b. Bring the victim to a sitting position.

    c. Have the victim lying on his or her back beside you.

    d. Place the victim on his side, arms extended over his or her head.

13. Which is a potential problem for a rescuer using the clothes drag?

    a. Back strain

    b. Wrist dislocation

    c. Bruised forearms

    d. Hernia

Objective 5

14. The two-person seat carry is appropriate for supporting the head and neck of a suspected spinal injury victim.

    T—[F]

15. A victim has jumped from the second story of a burning building and is lying on the ground. She has a laceration on her forehead and is barely conscious. You decide you must move her prior to providing first aid care. A second rescuer is with you. What would be the most appropriate emergency move for you to use with this victim?

    a. Walking assist

    b. Two-person seat carry

    c. Fireman's carry

    d. Clothes drag

16. The foot drag should not be used with a victim who may have a head or spine injury.

    [T]—F

Objective 6

17. The three safest methods of rescuing a near-drowning victim are reaching, throwing, and swimming assists.

    T—[F]

18. You are standing in your street clothes on your neighbor's pool deck when you see him struggling in the water at the deep end of the pool. What should you do to reach him and pull him to the side of the pool?

    a. Crouch at the edge of the pool and extend your hand or foot to him.

    b. Remove your shoes, shirt, and pants and jump in to assist him to the side.

    c. Call for help and wade toward the deep end to reach him.

    d. Lie down at the side of the pool and reach to him with one of your arms.

19. Where should you aim to throw a ring buoy to assist a near-drowning victim?

    a. Just short of the victim, within grasping range

    b. Directly to the victim, as close as possible

    c. Just beyond the victim

    d. Alongside the victim

20. You decide to wade into the water to assist a near-drowning victim. You will have a better chance of success if you can reach the victim with your hand rather than with an object like a branch or pole.

T—[F]

Objective 7

21. Which type of shirt may trap air and be helpful in rescuing you from water?

  a. A loose-fitting T-shirt
  b. A short-sleeved shirt that buttons
  c. A long-sleeved sweatshirt
  d. A long-sleeved shirt that buttons

22. Which position do you take in the water for survival floating?

  a. Facedown
  b. On your back
  c. Treading water
  d. None of the above

23. In floating on your back for self-rescue, you should keep your arms close to your body and kick gently toward shore.

T—[F]

Objective 8

24. Which of the following should you do to increase your safety around water?

  a. Make sure you tell someone before you go swimming alone.
  b. If possible, walk barefoot on a slippery dock.
  c. Stay with at least one other person when near water.
  d. All of the above

25. You should keep a Coast Guard-approved personal flotation device (PFD) within reach whenever you and your family are working or playing around water.

[T]—F

Objective 9

26. Match each term on the right with its definition on the left. Put its letter on the line in front of the definition.

h	A facedown floating technique used in warm water to conserve energy while waiting for rescue	a.	Clothes drag
e	A situation in which a person who has been submerged in water survives	b.	Drowning
f	A buoyant device designed to be held or worn to keep an individual afloat	c.	Fireman's carry
c	A technique for moving a victim in which the victim lies across the rescuer's shoulders	d.	Foot drag
a	A one-person technique that is useful for moving a victim with head or spine injury	e.	Near-drowning
		f.	Personal flotation device (PFD)
		g.	Seat carry
		h.	Survival

Chapter 18—Your Guide to a Healthier Life

Objective 1

1. Which of the following should you eat more of to improve your diet?

  a. Carbohydrates
  b. Fats
  c. Fiber
  d. Salt

2. A healthy, well-balanced diet includes at least four servings of enriched whole-grain breads or cereals daily.

[T]—F

3. Reducing your intake of fats, sodium, and cholesterol is a way of improving your diet.

[T]—F

4. At a minimum, how many glasses of water should you drink daily?

   a. 4

   b. 6

   c. 8

   d. 10

5. Obesity increases health risks because of the accompanying—

   a. Excess of fluid.

   b. Excess of body fat.

   c. Excess of body weight.

   d. Excess of sugar in the blood.

6. To attain the most accurate measure of weight loss, you should weigh yourself daily.

   T—[F]

7. As a person grows older, the total number of calories in his or her daily diet should gradually increase.

   T—[F]

Objective 2

8. A 25-year-old is starting a cardiovascular fitness program. What Target Heart Rate (THR) should he or she seek to achieve during exercise?

   a. 108–126 beats per minute

   b. 127–156 beats per minute

   c. 146–175 beats per minute

   d. 165–195 beats per minute

9. How does cardiovascular fitness contribute to a healthier lifestyle?

   a. It reduces the level of sugar in the blood.

   b. It helps to ward off infections.

   c. It improves individual self-esteem.

   d. b and c

10. If you experience a small amount of pain during exercise, you are exercising strenuously enough to build cardiovascular fitness.

    T—[F]

11. One way to reduce stress is to avoid foods containing—

    a. Cholesterol.

    b. Sugar.

    c. Caffeine.

    d. Fats.

Objective 3

12. Smoking increases the risk of—

    I. Lung cancer.

    II. Diabetes.

    III. Heart attack.

    IV. Stomach ulcers.

    ---

    a. I and III

    b. II and IV

    c. I, II, and III

    d. All of the above

13. The danger to an unborn baby whose mother smokes comes from the—

    a. Lack of oxygen in the mother's blood.

    b. Carbon monoxide and nicotine in cigarettes.

    c. Rise in the mother's blood pressure.

    d. All of the above

14. Substituting chewing tobacco or snuff for cigarettes reduces a person's risk of developing cancer.

    T—[F]

Objective 4

15. To avoid reaching a blood alcohol level that impairs judgment and reflexes, you should limit yourself to—

    a. One drink per hour.

    b. Two drinks per hour.

    c. Three drinks per hour.

    d. Four drinks per hour.

16. Which of the following can you do to help keep the effects of alcohol consumption under control?

    a. Drink beer instead of wine or mixed drinks.

    b. Drink plenty of black coffee before driving after you have consumed alcohol.

    c. Do not drink when you are eating meals or snacks.

    d. Do not drink when you are angry or depressed.

17. A cold shower will help decrease the impaired judgment and coordination that results from alcohol consumption.

    T—[F]

Objective 5

18. Which of the following should you do to increase safety in your home?
    a. Keep firearms and ammunition together in a cabinet higher than your children can reach.
    b. Equip all stairways with handrails.
    c. Put locks on all upstairs windows.
    d. All of the above

19. As part of your home safety plan, you should check your heating and cooling systems annually before use.

    [T]—F

20. As part of your home safety plan, you should put all your firearms and ammunition in a single locked cabinet out of the reach of your children.

    T—[F]

Objective 6

21. Which elements should you include in a fire escape plan for your home?
    a. Identification of at least two ways to get out of each room
    b. Designation of who will search each room before leaving the house
    c. Location of the phone from which the fire department will be called
    d. a and c

22. Which is the safest way to escape from a burning building through a smoke-filled hall?
    a. Standing upright and running quickly through the hall
    b. Covering your face with a wet towel and walking at a normal pace
    c. Crawling to keep as close to the floor as possible
    d. Staying close to the side wall and carefully feeling your way

23. You are on the 11th floor of a hotel when the fire alarm sounds. You should leave your room and take the elevator to the lobby as quickly as possible.

    T—[F]

24. You are trapped in a room by smoke and fire. You should stuff the door cracks and vents with wet towels.

    [T]—F

Objective 7

25. Which do you need to know to increase your safety at work?
    a. The shortest route to the hospital
    b. The amount of hazardous materials in your building
    c. The location of the nearest fire extinguisher
    d. All of the above

26. The agency whose rules are intended to minimize hazards in the workplace is the—
    a. Food and Drug Administration.
    b. Occupational Safety and Health Administration.
    c. National Institutes of Health.
    d. National Association of Manufacturers.

27. To increase your safety at work, you should make certain that you are informed of the actions you should take in case of a fire in your building.

    [T]—F

Objective 8

28. The best way to avoid being injured in a motor vehicle crash is to—
    a. Avoid drinking and driving.
    b. Always obey the speed limit.
    c. Always wear your safety belt.
    d. Avoid driving when you are tired.

29. All 50 states and the District of Columbia require a motorist to use a child safety seat when transporting an infant.

    [T]—F

Objective 9

30. When purchasing a bicycle helmet, what organization's approval would you look for?

    I. American Bicycle Association

    II. Snell Memorial Foundation

    III. Underwriters Laboratories

    IV. American Society for Testing and Materials

    V. American National Standards Institute

    ---

    a. I or III

    b. III or IV

    c. II or IV

    d. II or V

31. Even if you are not playing in competitive tournaments, you should wear protective goggles when playing racquetball.

    [T]—F

32. Most drownings happen to people who are engaged in water sports such as swimming and diving.

    T—[F]

33. The leading cause of injury to older adults is motor vehicle crashes.

    T—[F]

Appendix D

American Red Cross First Aid—Responding to Emergencies Course Evaluation

We would like to know what you thought about this American Red Cross First Aid—Responding to Emergencies course. Please complete this evaluation.

1. Tell us what you thought of the course. (Circle or check your choice.)

	Strongly Agree	Agree	Not Sure	Dis- agree	Strongly Disagree	Did Not Use
a. The textbook explained things clearly.	1	2	3	4	5	❑
b. The skill sheets helped me understand the correct steps to take in an emergency.	1	2	3	4	5	❑
c. The videos helped me understand how I could use my skills in certain emergencies.	1	2	3	4	5	❑
d. The demonstrations in the videos were clear and helpful.	1	2	3	4	5	❑
e. The sidebars in the textbook were interesting and relevant.	1	2	3	4	5	❑
f. The application questions in the textbook helped me to apply the information.	1	2	3	4	5	❑
g. The study questions in the textbook helped me to understand, remember, and review the information.	1	2	3	4	5	❑
h. The overhead transparences reinforced the content.	1	2	3	4	5	❑
i. The instructor-led scenarios helped me to become confident about applying my skills and knowledge.	1	2	3	4	5	
j. I have confidence that I can do these skills correctly.	1	2	3	4	5	
k. The instructor was well prepared.	1	2	3	4	5	
l. The instructor gave clear instructions on what to do next.	1	2	3	4	5	
m. The instructor answered questions clearly.	1	2	3	4	5	
n. The instructor helped me during the practice sessions.	1	2	3	4	5	
o. I would recommend this course to a friend.	1	2	3	4	5	
p. I know when to use the skills I learned in this course.	1	2	3	4	5	
q. I had to work hard to pass this course.	1	2	3	4	5	

2. Was all the equipment in good order? ❑ Yes ❑ No
3. Was the classroom clean and comfortable? ❑ Yes ❑ No
4. Was the facility well suited to skill practice? ❑ Yes ❑ No
5. Did you have enough time to read? ❑ Yes ❑ No
6. Did you have enough time to practice? ❑ Yes ❑ No
7. Did you take this course to fulfill an academic requirement? ❑ Yes ❑ No

   If not, why did you take this course?

   ____

   ____

8. Did you learn what you wanted to learn? ❑ Yes ❑ No

   If yes, please specify:

   ____

   ____

   If no, what else did you want to learn?

   ____

   ____

9. What was your age at your last birthday? ________
10. Please check the highest level of education you have completed.

    ❑ Junior high school ❑ High school ❑ 1st year college ❑ Graduate school

    ❑ 2nd year college ❑ 3rd year college ❑ 4th year college ❑ Other (please specify): ________

11. How did you hear about this course?

    ❑ College catalog ❑ Newspaper ❑ Television ❑ Radio

    ❑ Friend or relative ❑ Employer ❑ Pamphlet or poster

    ❑ Other (please specify): ______________________________

12. Are you: ❑ Male ❑ Female
13. Do you have any other comments about this course or your instructor that you would like to share with us?

    ____

    ____

Thank you for answering these questions. We hope you enjoyed the course.

Appendix E

American Red Cross
First Aid—Responding to Emergencies
Instructor Evaluation

To continue to improve this First Aid—Responding to Emergencies course, the American Red Cross needs your help. Please complete the following evaluation form the **FIRST** time you teach this course. Detach and return the completed evaluation (either as a self-fold-and-seal mailer, or by placing a copy in an envelope) to—

American Red Cross
National Headquarters
Health and Safety Course Evaluations
17th and D Streets, N.W.
Washington, DC 20006

We also invite you to share any observations that you may have about the course at any time by completing another evaluation or by writing to the above address.

American Red Cross First Aid—Responding to Emergencies Instructor Evaluation

Background

1. Course completion date __/__/__/

2. I taught a:
   ❑ First Aid—Responding to Emergencies course
   ❑ First Aid—Responding to Emergencies Challenge
   ❑ First Aid—Responding to Emergencies Review Course

3. Is this your first time teaching this course? ❑ Yes ❑ No

   If no, how many times have you taught this course? ______

4. Total time required to complete the course: _____hours

5. Total number of participants:
   # passed ______ # failed ______

6. Number of sessions in this course:______

7. How would you describe the participants in this course?
   ❑ Mostly under age 18
   ❑ Mostly ages 18 to 40
   ❑ Mostly ages 41 to 65
   ❑ Mixed ages

8. In what setting did you teach this course?
   ❑ Work Site ❑ College (2 yr.)
   ❑ High School ❑ College (4 yr.)
   ❑ Red Cross Unit Building
   ❑ Other (describe)

   ____

9. Do you have current Red Cross authorization to teach this course?
   ❑ Yes ❑ No

10. How long have you been an American Red Cross First Aid—Responding to Emergencies instructor?

    ____

11. When you taught this course, which of the following did you use?
    ❑ Textbook ❑ Instructor's Manual
    ❑ Skill Sheets ❑ American Red Cross Course Video
    ❑ Color Transparencies ❑ Transparency Masters
    ❑ Computerized Test Bank

12. List any additional materials used to teach this course.

13. List any additional audiovisuals used to teach this course.

14. List any questions about the course that are not answered in the *Instructor's Manual.*

15. List any suggestions for improving the *Instructor's Manual.*

over

Optional: If you are willing to discuss your comments with us, please give us your name and a daytime phone number. We would like to be able to call you if we have any questions.

Name ________________________ Phone number (   ) ________________

________________________ ____________ ____ ______
Your mailing address City State Zip + 4

Red Cross unit name ________________________
(if applicable)

If one is developed, would you like to receive a national newsletter for instructors?
If yes, please check box ❑

—Fold here first—

—Tape closed here after second fold—

16. List any suggestions for improving the textbook.

17. List any suggestions for improving the course video and color transparencies.

18. List any suggestions for additional course aids you feel would improve your presentation of this course.

Thank you for taking the time to answer these questions. If you have any additional comments about the course, please include them on a separate sheet and include it with this evaluation.

—Fold here second—

RTE IM
1/91

____
____
____

Stamp

American Red Cross
National Headquarters
Health and Safety Course Evaluations
17th & D Streets, N.W.
Washington, DC 20006

American Red Cross First Aid—Responding to Emergencies Instructor Evaluation

Background

1. Course completion date __/__/__/
2. I taught a:
   - ❑ First Aid—Responding to Emergencies course
   - ❑ First Aid—Responding to Emergencies Challenge
   - ❑ First Aid—Responding to Emergencies Review Course
3. Is this your first time teaching this course? ❑ Yes ❑ No

   If no, how many times have you taught this course? ______
4. Total time required to complete the course: _____hours
5. Total number of participants:
   # passed ______ # failed ______
6. Number of sessions in this course: ______
7. How would you describe the participants in this course?
   - ❑ Mostly under age 18
   - ❑ Mostly ages 18 to 40
   - ❑ Mostly ages 41 to 65
   - ❑ Mixed ages
8. In what setting did you teach this course?
   - ❑ Work Site
   - ❑ College (2 yr.)
   - ❑ High School
   - ❑ College (4 yr.)
   - ❑ Red Cross Unit Building
   - ❑ Other (describe)

   ____

9. Do you have current Red Cross authorization to teach this course?
   ❑ Yes ❑ No
10. How long have you been an American Red Cross First Aid—Responding to Emergencies instructor?

    ____
11. When you taught this course, which of the following did you use?
    - ❑ Textbook
    - ❑ Instructor's Manual
    - ❑ Skill Sheets
    - ❑ American Red Cross Course Video
    - ❑ Color Transparencies
    - ❑ Transparency Masters
    - ❑ Computerized Test Bank
12. List any additional materials used to teach this course.
13. List any additional audiovisuals used to teach this course.
14. List any questions about the course that are not answered in the *Instructor's Manual.*
15. List any suggestions for improving the *Instructor's Manual.*

over

Optional: If you are willing to discuss your comments with us, please give us your name and a daytime phone number. We would like to be able to call you if we have any questions.

Name ______________________ Phone number (   ) ______________

______________________ ______________ ______ ______
Your mailing address City State Zip + 4

Red Cross unit name ______________________
(if applicable)

If one is developed, would you like to receive a national newsletter for instructors? If yes, please check box ❑

—Fold here first—

—Tape closed here after second fold—

16. List any suggestions for improving the textbook.

17. List any suggestions for improving the course video and color transparencies.

18. List any suggestions for additional course aids you feel would improve your presentation of this course.

Thank you for taking the time to answer these questions. If you have any additional comments about the course, please include them on a separate sheet and include it with this evaluation.

—Fold here second—

RTE IM
1/91

Stamp

American Red Cross
National Headquarters
Health and Safety Course Evaluations
17th & D Streets, N.W.
Washington, DC 20006

Appendix F

Use of Instructor Aides

Instructor aides can help you with some parts of the course and may help you use class time more efficiently. Instructor aides should have already completed the course in which they will be assisting. They may be individuals who have expressed an interest in becoming instructors.

It is your responsibility to ensure that instructor aides who assist with the class are trained. Before allowing an instructor aide to assist you, ask to see the aide's Instructor Aide Certificate (Certificate 3003) and current course completion certificates for the following American Red Cross courses:

- First Aid—Responding to Emergencies, and
- Adult CPR (or equivalent, issued within one year).

The duties and responsibilities of instructor aides will vary, depending on the aide's experience and ability. These duties should be limited to—

- Handling registration and record keeping.
- Setting up the classrooms and handing out supplies.
- Assisting with equipment (for example, setting up the VCR or cleaning manikins).
- Helping participants with practice activities (for example, finding practice partners).
- Scoring written exams.

Instructor aides may help participants during the practice sessions. Before allowing this, however, make sure that the aide can demonstrate the skills correctly and coach participants effectively.

Training of Instructor Aides

Contact your local Red Cross unit to obtain specific information regarding the training program for instructor aides. Aide training includes discussion of—

- Course objectives, both knowledge objectives (what the participant needs to know to pass the written test) and skill objectives (what the participant needs to know to pass the skills checks).
- Course materials and their use.
- Course administration and scheduling.
- Procedures for practice sessions.
- Relative responsibilities of the instructor and the aide.

Appendix G

Equipment Checklist

The following is a list of the equipment and materials needed to teach the American Red Cross First Aid—Responding to Emergencies course.

For the class:

- Viewing equipment: 1/2" VCR and monitor, overhead projector
- Extension cord and grounded plug adaptor, if needed
- Video: *American Red Cross First Aid—Responding to Emergencies* (Stock No. 650018)
- Decontamination supplies (decontaminating solution, 4" x 4" gauze pads, soap and water, baby bottle brush, basins or buckets, nonsterile disposable gloves, and any accessories that may be recommended by the manufacturer of the manikin)
- Chalkboard, chalk, and eraser, or
- Flip chart and marker pens, easel or tape
- Adult manikins (one for every two or three participants)

For participants:

- Name tags
- Pencils and/or pens
- Behavior Modification Contracts
- Participant Course Evaluations (Appendix D)
- Written examinations and blank answer sheets (Appendix B)
- Copies of alternate examination (Appendix B)
- *American Red Cross First Aid—Responding to Emergencies* textbook (Stock No. 650005)
- Blankets or mats (one for every two or three participants)
- Manikin decontamination supplies:
  - alcohol wipes or decontaminating solution and gauze pads
- External bleeding control materials:
  - 2 three-inch roller bandages for each participant
  - 4 nonsterile dressings or gauze pads for each participant
- Splinting materials for each pair of participants:
  - 5 triangular bandages
  - 1 three-inch roller bandage
  - Blanket or pillow
  - Rigid splint (magazine, cardboard, or board)

For the instructor:

- American Red Cross identification
- Name tag
- *American Red Cross First Aid—Responding to Emergencies* textbook (Stock No. 650005)
- *American Red Cross First Aid—Responding to Emergencies Instructor's Manual* (Stock No. 650010)
- Instructor Evaluation (Appendix E)
- Answer keys for both written exams (Appendix B) and scoring keys for both written exams (back of this manual)
- Extra manikin lungs
- *Course Record* (Form 6418) and *Course Record Addendum* (Form 6418A)
- Extra pens or pencils

Course Materials by Unit

Lesson Plan	Unit	Video	Needed	Transparency*
	Parts I through III			
1	Course Introduction		None	
2	Healthy Lifestyles		Behavior Modification Contract	TM 1 and 2
3	The Citizen Responder	✓	None	
4	Responding to Emergencies	✓	None	CT 1 through 3, TM 3 and 4
5	Body Systems	✓	None	CT 4 through 14
6	Primary/Secondary Survey I	✓	Blankets or mats Skill sheet Participant Progress Log	TM 5
7	Primary/Secondary Survey II	✓	Blankets or mat Skill sheet Participant Progress Log	TM 6
8	Respiratory Emergencies I		None	CT 5 through 7 TM 7 through 9
9	Respiratory Emergencies II	✓	Blankets or mats Skill sheet Adult manikins Decontamination supplies Participant Progress Log	TM 10
10	Respiratory Emergencies III (First Aid for an Obstructed Airway, Conscious and Unconscious)	✓	Blankets or mats Skill sheets Adult manikins Decontamination supplies Participant Progress Log	TM 11
11	Cardiac Emergencies I	✓	None	CT 8, 15 through 17 TM 12 and 13

*TM = Transparency Master
CT = Color Transparency

Lesson Plan	Unit	Video	Needed	Transparency*
12	Cardiac Emergencies II	✓	Blankets or mats Adult manikins Decontamination supplies	CT 16 through 18 TM 12 and 14
13	Cardiac Emergencies III		Blankets or mats Participant Progress Log Skill sheet Adult manikins Decontamination supplies	
14	Bleeding and Shock	✓	Roller bandages Gauze pads	CT 19 and 20 TM 15 through 21
15	Putting It All Together I		Blankets or mats Adult manikins and decontamination supplies (optional) Self-assessment exercise 1	TM 1, 22 through 26
16	Putting It All Together II		Blankets or mats Adult manikins and decontamination supplies (optional) Self-assessment exercise 1 and answer key	TM 22 through 26

Lesson Plan	Unit	Video	Needed	Transparency*
	Part IV			
17	Injuries	✓	Healthy Lifestyles Awareness Inventory	CT 1 TM 27 though 29
18	Soft Tissue Injuries I	✓	Blankets or mats Gauze pads Roller bandages Skill sheets Participant Progress Log	CT 21 through 24 TM 30
19	Soft Tissue Injuries II/ Musculoskeletal Injuries I	✓	None	CT 10 through 13, 25 through 36 TM 31 through 33
20	Musculoskeletal Injuries II		Blankets Triangular bandagess Rigid splints Participant Progress Log Skill sheets	
21	Specific Injuries		None	CT 36 thtough 42 TM 24 through 38
22	Putting It All Together I		Blankets or mats Manikins (optional) Various splinting devices Triangular bandages Roller gauze Self-assessment exercise 2	CT 1 TM 26, 39 through 41
23	Putting It All Together II		Blankets or mats Manikins (optional) Various splinting devices Triangular bandages Roller gauze Gauze pads Self-assessment exercise 2 and answer key	CT 1 TM 26, 39 through 41

Lesson Plan	Unit	Video	Needed	Transparency*
	Part V			
24	Medical Emergencies	✓	None	CT 43 through 47 TM 42 through 49
25	Substance Misuse and Abuse		None	TM 50 and 51
26	Heat and Cold Exposure		Self-assessment exercise 3	CT 48 TM 26, 52 through 60
27	Putting It All Together		Blankets or mats Adult manikins and decontamination supplies (optional) Self-assessment exercise 3 and answer key	TM 26, 58 through 60
	Part VI			
28	Rescue Moves	✓	None	TM 26, and 61 through 65
	Part VII			
29	Your Guide to a Healthy Lifestyle		None	TM 66 through 68
	Part VIII			
30	Reviewing the Course		Blankets or mats Bandaging and splinting equipment or supplies Adult manikins and decontamination supplies (optional)	TM 69 and 70
31	Final Written Examination		Final examinations Answer sheets Answer key Scoring key Course evaluations	

Appendix I

Common "Critical" Errors Made During Practice Sessions

The following list of common "critical" errors will help you when you are watching participants work through the practice sessions.

Primary Survey

Kneeling too far away from the victim's body instead of right next to the victim

Skipping the check for unresponsiveness

Neglecting to shout for help

When opening the airway, placing one hand on the victim's forehead and the other beneath the neck

When opening the airway, placing one hand under the neck and the other under the chin

When opening the airway, not tilting the head back far enough

When opening the airway, applying pressure to the soft part of the throat when lifting the chin

When checking for breathlessness, checking for only about 1 second

When checking for breathlessness, looking in the opposite direction, away from the chest

When giving 2 full breaths, not tilting the head back far enough to maintain an open airway

Not getting the manikin's chest to rise when giving breaths

When giving 2 full breaths, neglecting to pinch the nose shut

When checking for pulse, feeling the pulse for only about 1 second

After checking for pulse, neglecting to say whether there is a pulse present

Neglecting to instruct a bystander to phone EMS for help

Secondary Survey

Failing to complete a primary survey before doing a secondary survey

Failing to get consent to care for the victim

Failing to interview the victim properly by not asking key questions

When checking the radial pulse, placing the fingers in the wrong location, or using the thumb

Failing to realize that pulse or breathing rate is above or below normal

Failing to recognize that a possible serious injury has occurred and manipulating the victim's head and neck

Having the victim attempt to move an area the victim says is painful

Failing to check some body parts

Rescue Breathing

When giving rescue breaths, giving 1 breath every 5 seconds without maintaining an open airway

When giving rescue breaths, neglecting to pinch the nose shut

When giving rescue breaths, giving 1 breath every 2 or 3 seconds or every 7 to 9 seconds

First Aid for Complete Airway Obstruction, Unconscious Adult

Skipping the check for unresponsiveness

After giving 2 full breaths and the air has not gone in, forgetting to retilt the head and reattempt to give breaths

After retilting the head and giving the second set of 2 full breaths, neglecting to recognize that the airway is obstructed.

Neglecting to instruct a bystander to phone EMS for help

When giving abdominal thrusts, placing one hand against the lower edge of the victim's rib cage and the other hand directly on top of the first hand

When giving abdominal thrusts, using too much or too little pressure

Giving only 4 abdominal thrusts before doing a finger sweep

Failing to do a finger sweep

First Aid for Complete Airway Obstruction, Conscious Adult

Neglecting to ask the victim if he or she is choking

Neglecting to shout for help

When performing abdominal thrusts, wrapping the arms around the lower edge of the victim's rib cage

When performing abdominal thrusts, standing beside the victim rather than behind the victim

CPR

Rather than correctly locating the compression point, placing the hands directly over the breastbone without feeling for appropriate landmarks (lower edge of rib cage; notch)

When giving chest compressions, placing the hands too high or too low on the breastbone

When giving chest compressions, compressing the breastbone less than 1 inch

When giving chest compressions, bending the elbows with each compression

When giving chest compressions, compressing too fast or too slowly

During CPR, giving 2 full breaths after every 5 compressions

When giving CPR, checking the pulse after 2 cycles of 15 compressions and 2 breaths

Neglecting to recheck the pulse

Controlling External Bleeding

Failing to apply direct pressure

Failing to apply a dressing before bandaging

Failing to anchor the bandage securely before wrapping

Wrapping the bandage too loosely

Failing to elevate the wound above the level of the heart

When locating the pressure points, placing the hand in the wrong position

Splinting

Neglecting to immobilize the joints above and below the fracture site

Neglecting to check circulation by checking color and temperature of a limb before splinting

Putting the splint on top of the fracture site

Tying cravats over the fracture site

Not padding the knots

Failing to recheck circulation after splinting

Physically Challenged Participants

As an American Red Cross First Aid—Responding to Emergencies instructor, you may be asked to present this course to a class that includes one or more physically challenged participants. Physically challenged individuals include those who are hearing or sight-impaired, lack full use of limbs, have breathing difficulties, or other physical problems. In some instances, entire classes may be composed of this special group. When the physically challenged individual can meet the stated course objectives, he or she can, and should, receive the course completion certificates.

This section does not provide detailed instructions on how to modify the material to accommodate specific impairments; rather, it provides a series of considerations that are likely to provide a successful outcome. Whenever you help the participant during the learning process, you must ensure that the participant is able to meet the course objectives without aid during skill checks. Participants who cannot perform the skills have not met the course objectives and cannot receive national course completion certificates.

Key Points

- Physically challenged individuals **can** learn first aid skills and CPR.
- Instructors must learn to adapt their teaching to these individuals.
- Instructors must retain the guidelines, objectives, and policies that describe a particular skill.
- There is no one strategy for teaching participants who have physical limitations.
- Methods of recognizing the limitations include—
  - Instructor observation of participants.
  - Participants' statements.
- Some first aid skills require strenuous effort. Be alert to participants who are in poor physical condition or have medical problems.

How to Help the Participant Overcome Physical Challenges

As the instructor, you may modify the delivery of course material in the following manner:
- Increase the amount of time you spend with each participant.
- Allow frequent rests.

- Help participants modify the techniques necessary for successful skill completion. For example, a participant with one arm could be instructed to seal the nose with his or her cheek while using his or her arm and hand to do the head-tilt/chin-lift skill in rescue breathing.

Emphasize the value of information and skills learned, regardless of whether or not participants can be awarded course completion certificates.

Appendix K
Participant Progress Log

Instructor: ______________________ **Course Date and Time:** ______________________

Place a check (✓) in the appropriate space after a participant completes each skill check and passes the written test.

	Skills										
Name of Participant	**Positioning the Victim**	**Primary Survey**	**Secondary Survey**	**Rescue Breathing**	**Choking/ Unconscious Adult**	**Choking/ Conscious Adult**	**Adult CPR**	**Control of Bleeding**	**Splinting**	**Written Test**	**Comments**
1.											
2.											
3.											
4.											
5.											
6.											
7.											
8.											
9.											
10.											

Appendix L

Instructor Self-Assessment and Development

Instructors: Using the assessment categories (A,B,C, and D) described below, rate yourself as well as you can on each of the following instructor skills.

A — Little or no experience in this
B — Some experience but uncertain degree of skill
C — Some skill
D — Good skill

A	B	C	D	Instruction Skills
				1. Planning and managing physical environment (tables, seating, lighting, audiovisual aids, papers)
				2. Setting and maintaining an effective learning climate
				3. Interpreting, applying, and presenting textbook material
				4. Assigning tasks and giving instructions clearly and concisely
				5. Adjusting to group and individual response, and stimulating participation as needed
				6. Managing time
				7. Being able to interpret and implement a Red Cross course design, involving the integration of course content, method, and materials
				8. Evaluating participants' achievement of the course learning objectives
				9. Summarizing material
				10. Maintaining the kind of class discussion that facilitates learning
				11. Bridging effectively—moving from one topic to another
				12. Wrapping up and being conscious of vantage points in the course, summarizing those points
				13. Being aware of my personal image—attributes that add or detract from my other instructor skills

For other self-development, prepare a developing planning worksheet, to include—

OBJECTIVES	PLAN FOR ACCOMPLSHING	RESOURCES

Appendix M

Guidelines for Conducting American Red Cross First Aid—Responding to Emergencies Reviews

The American Red Cross First Aid—Responding to Emergencies Review has two formats: (1) a challenge format and (2) a review course that is an abbreviated version of the original course. For either format, the instructor must be an authorized American Red Cross First Aid—Responding to Emergencies instructor. To be eligible for the challenge or the review course, the participant must—

- Possess an American Red Cross First Aid—Responding to Emergencies certificate (653215), issued within three years, and
- Possess an American Red Cross: Adult CPR certificate (C-3212) or equivalent, issued within one year.

Length

The length of the challenge and the review course will be determined by the instructor and will vary depending on several factors, including—

- Number of participants.
- Number of manikins used.
- Experience of instructor.
- Time since previous training.
- Amount of coaching or practice time needed.

OPTION 1

Challenge

The purpose is to provide individuals the opportunity to prove their knowledge and competencies in specific skills. Participants should be informed of this responsibility prior to the challenge session. All responsibility for preparedness for the challenge rests solely on the participants. Your responsibility is to assess and verify the participants' knowledge and competency.

In order to challenge the American Red Cross First Aid—Responding to Emergencies course, the participant must do the following in the following order:

- Pass a 70-question written examination with a score of 80 percent or higher. (See Appendix B of the *American Red Cross First Aid—Responding to Emergencies Instructor's Manual.)*
- Successfully demonstrate the following skills: (See Participant Progress Log, Appendix K of the *American Red Cross First Aid—Responding to Emergencies Instructor's Manual.)*
  - Positioning the victim
  - Primary survey
  - Secondary survey
  - Rescue breathing
  - Obstructed airway—conscious and unconscious adult

- Adult CPR
- Controlling bleeding
- Splinting

OPTION 2

Review Course

The purpose of the review course is to provide individuals with an opportunity to review the material within a formal course structure. The responsibility for preparing for the final exam and skills checks is shared by the instructor and the participant. (The participant must be notified that he or she is responsible for reviewing contents of the textbook either prior to the class or as homework.)

The outline for this review course, on page 329, is based on the lesson plans in this manual.

By the end of the review course, the participants must—

- Pass a 70-question written examination from Appendix B in the instructor's manual.
- Successfully complete the skill checks as described in the Challenge Format.

Certification and Recordkeeping—Challenge and Review Course

Prepare *Course Record* (Form 6418) and, if needed, *Course Record Addendum* (Form 6418A) and indicate American Red Cross First Aid—Responding to Emergencies Review (Course Code 3215R) for submission to the Red Cross unit.

Issue or mail course completion certificates for both American Red Cross: Adult CPR and American Red Cross First Aid—Responding to Emergencies to participants who have successfully completed either format of the review.

American Red Cross First Aid—Responding to Emergencies Review Course Outline

Lesson	Content	Activity	Prior Reading Assignment	Video
1	Introduction to Course, The Citizen Responder, Responding to Emergencies	Discussion, Primary Points	Preface, About this Course, Ch. 1 and 3	✔
2	Body Systems, Bleeding and Shock	Discussion, Primary Points	Ch. 2, 6 and 7	✔
3	Primary/Secondary Survey I	Skill Practice: Primary Survey		✔
4	Primary/Secondary Survey II	Skill Practice: Secondary Survey	Ch. 4	✔
5	Respiratory Emergencies I	Discussion, Skill Practice: Rescue Breathing		✔
6	Respiratory Emergencies II	Skill Practice: Obstructed Airway		✔
7	Cardiac Emergencies I	Discussion, Skill Practice: CPR	Ch. 5	✔
8	Cardiac Emergencies II	Skill Practice: CPR		
9	Soft Tissue Injuries	Skill Practice: Controlling Bleeding	Ch. 8	✔
10	Musculoskeletal Injuries	Discussion, Skill Practice: Immobilization	Ch. 9, 10, 11, 12	✔
11	Medical Emergencies, Substance Misuse and Abuse	Discussion, Primary Points	Ch. 13, 14, 15	✔
12	Heat and Cold Exposure, Rescue Moves, Your Guide to a Healthier Life	Discussion, Primary Points	Ch. 16, 17, 18	
13	Reviewing the Course	Discussion, Scenarios		
14	Final Written Examination	Examination, Evaluation		

Total Course Time ***approximately 10 hours, 30 minutes***

Appendix N

Behavior Modification Contract

Now that you have taken the time to evaluate your lifestyle, you may be able to identify behaviors that could lead to injury or illness, now or in the future. Identifying these behaviors is the first step to leading a healthier life. By using this contract as a tool, it will help you focus on working toward one specific goal to make your lifestyle healthier.

Goal: Complete the sentence below. Be as specific as you can.

In the ____weeks of this course, my goal is to—

Objectives: Make a list of the lifestyle changes that are necessary to accomplish your goal. For instance, if your goal is to lose 10 pounds, you might want to make these changes in lifestyle: to lower the fat intake in your diet, exercise at least three times a week, and start eating a nutritious breakfast daily.

1.
2.
3.
4.
5.

Evaluation: To realize your goals, it is important to measure your progress at regular intervals. Make a list of the ways in which you will track your progress.

1.
2.
3.
4.
5.

Reward: Rewarding positive changes in behavior is important. When I meet my goal, I will reward myself by—

I agree to do my best to accomplish the goal of this contract during the time allotted.

Name ____

Date ____

Witness ____

This is only one step in your quest to lead a healthier life. Once you have reached this goal, continue to set others, as you feel may be necessary. A healthy lifestyle is a lifetime of healthy behaviors.

Appendix O

Administrative Terms and Procedures

For further information on any of the following terms and procedures, ask your Instructor Trainer or contact your local Red Cross unit.

Instructor—A member of a select group of individuals authorized to serve as agents of the Red Cross by teaching American Red Cross basic courses and imparting knowledge and skills consistent with American Red Cross policies, procedures, standards, and guidelines.

Red Cross Unit—Any Red Cross chapter, field service territory, or SAF station.

Certified—Receipt of a completion certificate when a participant has met all minimum course requirements of a Red Cross course.

Authorized—To be accepted by a local Red Cross unit to teach a Red Cross course in that unit's jurisdiction. To become authorized, the Health and Safety Instructor Certificate (Form 5736) and the Instructor Agreement (Form 6574) must be signed by you and a Red Cross unit official from your unit of authorization.

Reauthorization—The act of being authorized again by teaching or co-teaching at least one First Aid—Responding to Emergencies course during your authorization period. You will receive a Health and Safety Instructor Authorization certificate (C-3005) when you are reauthorized.

Extended Authorization—When you wish to teach on a temporary basis within another Red Cross unit's jurisdiction, you must contact that unit to get your instructor certificate endorsed for extended authorization. You must also notify that unit prior to any teaching activity and observe any procedures specific to that unit.

Transfer of Authorization—If you relocate for any reason, your authorization may be accepted by the Red Cross unit in your new jurisdiction. Contact your new Red Cross unit for further information on how the Red Cross can transfer your teaching records to your new location.

Suspension/Withdrawal of Authorization—The local Red Cross unit grants an Instructor authorization to teach. It is also the Red Cross unit's responsibility to suspend or withdraw the Instructor authorization for due cause. Due cause, generally, means that the Instructor does not or will not abide by the standards, policies, or procedures of the Red Cross organization and its programs or in some way abuses the position of an authorized Red Cross Instructor.

Teaching Records—Your Red Cross unit of authorization maintains your teaching and training records for the purpose of reauthorization, awards, and recognition, etc.

Course of Record—A course for which a properly completed, duly signed Course Record (Form 6418) and, if necessary, a Course Record Addendum (Form 6418A) have been submitted to and accepted by a Red Cross unit in the jurisdiction in which the course was conducted.

Minimum Enrollment for Courses—Each course must have enough participants to provide course participants with sufficient skill practice to accomplish the course objectives. Therefore, you must obtain prior permission from your local Red Cross to conduct a course with fewer than six participants. Courses must have a minimum of six participants enrolled, not necessarily passing.

Co-Teach—To share full or 100 percent participation in course leadership with one or more co-instructors. Co-teaching is also known as team teaching.

Instructor Aide—An individual who successfully completes instructor aide training to help an instructor with a basic course.

Instructor Agreement (Form 6574)—A form signed by Red Cross instructors before being authorized to teach a Red Cross course. It explains the rights and responsibilities of both the instructor and the Red Cross unit of authorization.

Appendix P

Color Transparencies

This appendix contains a list of color transparencies that are available as a separate stock item (650012). These transparencies may be used to support class discussion and activities as you wish. Appendix G, Equipment Checklist, provides a quick reference to the transparencies appropriate for each lesson.

Color Transparencies

1 Emergency Action Principles

2 The Citizen Responder

3 The Chain of Survival

4 Cells, Tissues, and Organs

5 The Respiratory System

6 The Lungs

7 The Breathing Process

8 The Heart

9 The Nervous System

10 The Bones of the Musculoskeletal System

11 A Joint

12 The Muscles of the Musculoskeletal System

13 Muscle Movement

14 The Integumentary System

15 The Chest

16 Coronary Arteries and Coronary Artery Disease

17 Signals of a Heart Attack

18 Adult, Child, Infant CPR

19 Blood Loss

20 Signals of Shock

21 Skin Cross Section
Bruise

22 Abrasion
Laceration

23 Avulsion
Puncture Wound

24 Impaled Object
Infection

25 Skin Cross Section
Superficial Burn

26 Partial-Thickness Burn
Full-Thickness Burn

27 Muscle Contraction

28 The Chest
The Skull

29 Similarities of Bones

30 Types of Bones

31 Joint Motion

32 The Skeleton—Parts of the Body

33 Fracture
Dislocation

34 Sprain
Strain

35 Sprain and Strain Sites

36 Splinting

37 Common Causes of Spine Injury

38 The Spine

39 The Chest
The Abdomen

40 Sucking Chest Wound

41 The Pelvis

42 Shoulder Injuries

43 Signals of a Medical Emergency

44 Diabetic Emergencies

45 Stroke

46 Poisoning

47 Poison Control Center

48 Adjusting to Heat and Cold

Appendix Q

Transparency Masters

This appendix includes 70 transparency masters which may be used to support class discussion and activities as you wish to do so. Appropriate use of each transparency master is included as part of the lesson plans. Appendix G, Equipment Checklist, provides a quick reference to the transparencies needed for each lesson.

Many of the transparency masters are suitable for use as handouts.

Transparency Masters

KEY TO MODIFYING BEHAVIOR

- Want to change
- Change attitudes
- Maintain changed attitudes

TM2

BEHAVIOR MODIFICATION STRATEGIES

- Evaluate present behaviors.
- Decide behaviors to change.
- Set goals.
- Use rewards.
- Avoid situations that promote negative behavior.
- Reinforce commitment to change.
- Use the support of others.
- Seek professional help.

SCENARIO 1:

You see a car veer off the road, striking a utility pole. The pole splinters, dropping wires on the vehicle. You decide to help. How would you respond?

SCENARIO 2:

You arrive at your grandfather's home and find him lying motionless in the backyard. You hear a neighbor in the yard next door. You decide to help. How would you respond?

SCENARIO 3:

While jogging, you notice a bike rider fall as she rounds a corner on a rain-slick road. With her crumpled bike nearby, she is lying in the road moaning. You decide to help. How would you respond?

SCENARIO 4:

During a softball game, a ball is hit between two players. Both converge on the ball. They collide, falling to the ground. One player is holding his arm, screaming in pain. The second player lies motionless. You decide to help. How would you respond?

KEY POINTS OF A PRIMARY SURVEY

- Check consciousness.
- Check ABCs — **A**irway.
  Breathing.
  Circulation.

KEY POINTS OF A SECONDARY SURVEY

- Interview the victim and bystanders.
- Check vital signs.
- Do a head-to-toe exam.

COMMON CAUSES OF RESPIRATORY DISTRESS

- Asthma
- Hyperventilation
- Anaphylactic Shock

TM8

RESPIRATORY DISTRESS

	Asthma	Hyperventilation	Anaphylactic Shock
Facts:	Narrowing of air passage makes breathing difficult More common in children Usually controlled by medication	Rapid breathing causes an upset in the body's balance of oxygen and carbon dioxide	Swelling of air passages restricts breathing Also known as anaphylaxis
Can be triggered by:	Allergic reaction to pollen, food, a drug, insect stings Emotional stress or physical activity	Fear/anxiety Injury to the head, severe bleeding, illness Asthma Exercise	Severe allergic reaction to food, insect stings, a drug
Signals:	Wheezing when exhaling	Shallow, rapid breathing Dizziness Numbness in fingers/toes	Skin rash Tightness in the chest/ throat Swelling of the face/neck/ tongue

CARING FOR RESPIRATORY DISTRESS

General Care —

- Emergency Action Principles

Specific Care —

- Place victim in a sitting position.
- Reduce heat/humidity.
- Provide fresh air.

TM10

KEY POINTS OF RESPIRATORY ARREST

- Life-threatening
- Breathing stops
- Often preceded by respiratory distress
- Body systems fail

AIRWAY OBSTRUCTION

Anatomical

Blocked by anatomic structure

- Tongue
- Swelling of throat

Mechanical

Blocked by foreign object

- Food
- Toy
- Fluid

TM12

CARING FOR A HEART ATTACK

- Stop activity.
- Rest in a comfortable position.
- Call EMS.
- Monitor vital signs.
- Monitor changes in appearance and behavior.
- Be calm and reassuring.

CONTROLLABLE RISK FACTORS OF CARDIOVASCULAR DISEASE

- Smoking
- Diet high in fat
- High blood pressure
- Obesity
- Lack of exercise

TM14

COMMON CAUSES OF CARDIAC ARREST

- Cardiovascular disease
- Drowning
- Suffocation
- Electrocution
- Poisoning
- Respiratory arrest
- Severe blood loss

THE CIRCULATORY SYSTEM

Heart **Blood** **Blood Vessels**

Blood:

Liquid (plasma)

Solid components (white and red blood cells, platelets)

Blood Vessels:

Arteries

Veins

Capillaries

TM16

MAJOR FUNCTIONS OF BLOOD

- Protect against disease
- Maintain constant body temperature
- Transport oxygen, nutrients, and wastes

SIGNALS OF EXTERNAL BLEEDING

Arterial	Often rapid, profuse Spurts from wound Difficult to control
Venous	Flows from wound at a steady rate
Capillary	Oozes from wound

TM18

CARING FOR EXTERNAL BLEEDING

- Direct pressure
- Elevation
- Pressure bandage

If necessary:

- Pressure point
- Call EMS

SIGNALS OF INTERNAL BLEEDING

- Discoloration
- Tender/swollen/hard tissues
- Anxiety/restlessness
- Rapid breathing
- Cool/moist/pale/bluish skin
- Nausea/vomiting
- Excessive thirst
- Declining level of consciousness

TM20

CARING FOR SHOCK

1) Follow EAPs.

2) Provide general care:

    Monitor ABCs.

    Do no further harm.

    Help the victim rest comfortably.

    Maintain normal body temperature.

    Reassure the victim.

3) Provide specific care:

    Control external bleeding.

    Elevate legs.

    Give nothing to eat/drink.

    Call EMS.

SCENARIO

You are hiking with a friend on a marked trail in a local park. You both decide to stray from this path in search of more challenging terrain. Your friend loses his footing on loose rocks and falls approximately 15 feet down the rocky incline. When you reach him, you notice that he is bleeding badly from a deep wound on the lower leg.

- How would you provide care?

In attempting to control bleeding, you raise your friend's leg. He cries out in pain.

- How do you react?
- Does your care change?

After several minutes have passed, you notice that your friend appears pale and is sweating. He tells you he is feeling a little dizzy and nauseated. He asks for water from your canteen.

- How do you respond?

TM22

SCENARIO 1

At work, you are summoned to assist a fellow worker who has been injured in a 5-foot fall from a ladder. As you arrive, you notice the person sitting on the ground, writhing in pain and having trouble breathing as he clutches his arm to his chest. You want to help. How do you proceed?

SCENARIO 2

A frantic neighbor is knocking at your door. She says that she cannot wake her sleeping roommate. She remembers that her roommate took some pills about two hours ago, but she is not sure what they were or where her roommate keeps them. You enter and see a woman lying face up on the couch but not moving. How do you proceed?

SCENARIO 3

It's early morning, and you are taking a swim. The pool is almost deserted. Only two other people are swimming. When you finish, you realize you have to hurry or be late for class. As you enter the locker room, you are startled to see a body lying motionless on the damp floor next to a row of lockers. You recognize the older person as one who had been swimming laps next to you. You want to help. How do you proceed?

SCENARIO 4

Awakened in the early morning by your mother's scream, you rush to your parents' bedroom. There you find your father lying motionless on the floor. Your mother tells you that he had been feeling ill for several hours and had vomited. She says that he emerged from the bathroom clutching his chest and in apparent pain. He suddenly collapsed to the floor. You want to help. How do you proceed?

SCENARIO 5

You witness a bicyclist struck by a car. The bicyclist is thrown from the bike, striking her head. The driver of the vehicle gets out to help. As you approach, you see the bicyclist lying on her side, twitching. Blood is spurting from the victim's thigh onto the pavement. You want to help. How do you proceed?

TM26

KEY TO PROVIDING CARE

Did the groups —

1) Follow the EAPs?
   - Survey the scene.
   - Do a primary survey.
   - Call EMS.
   - Do a secondary survey.
2) Involve bystanders appropriately?
3) Demonstrate proper care?

LEADING CAUSES OF INJURY-RELATED DEATHS, 1988

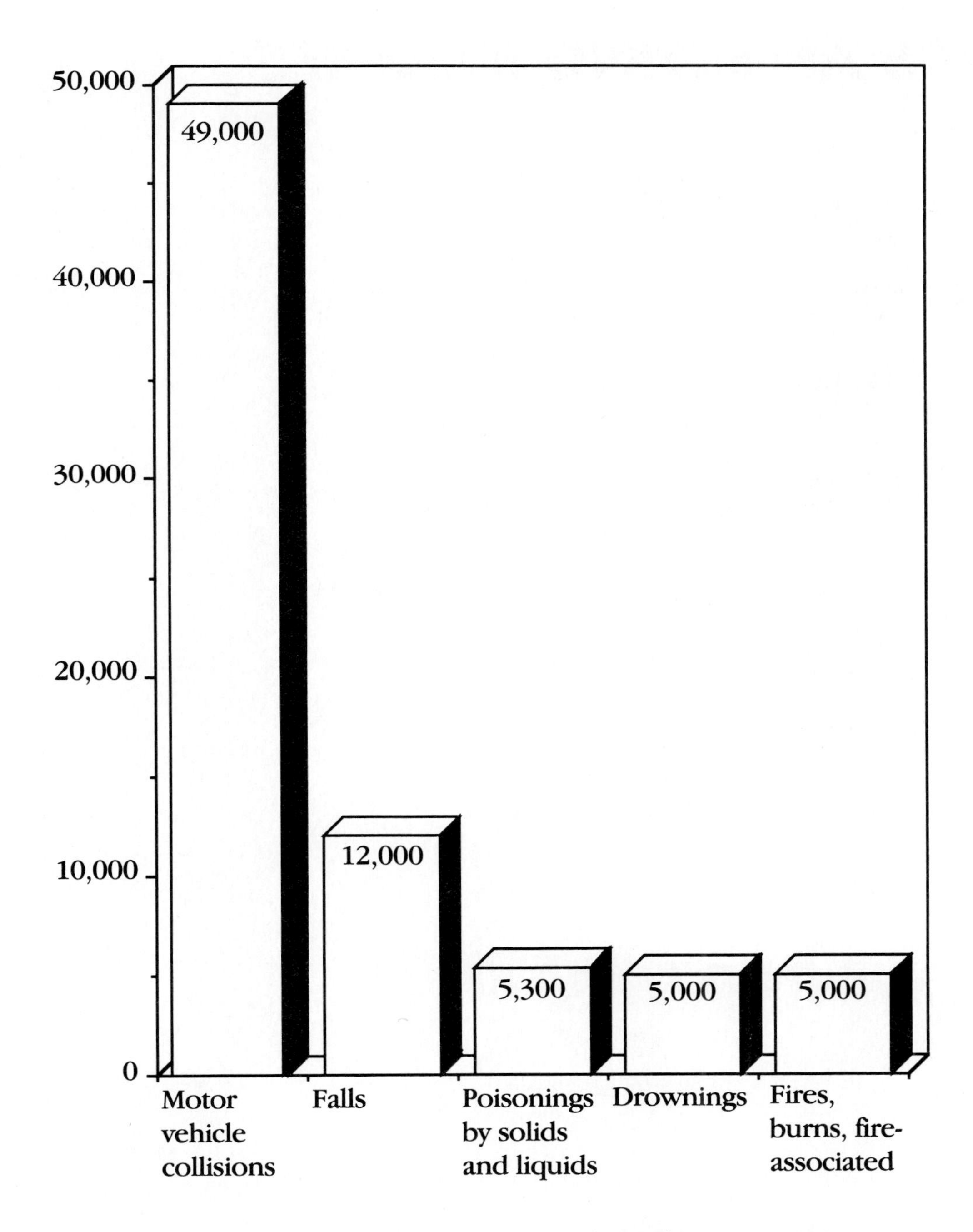

(Data from National Safety Council, *Accident Facts*, 1989)

FACTORS AFFECTING INJURIES

- Age
- Gender
- Environment
- Alcohol Use/Abuse

INJURY-PREVENTION STRATEGIES

Societal

- Alter behavior of people at risk.
- Require change by law.
- Provide automatic protection.

Personal

- Know your risks.
- Change your behaviors.
- Think safety.

CARING FOR WOUNDS

Closed Wound	Major Open Wound	Minor Open Wound
Direct pressure	**Do not** wash wound	Wash wound
Elevation	Apply clean dressing	Apply clean dressing
Cold	Direct pressure	Direct pressure
Seek medical attention if severe injury is suspected	Elevation	Antibiotic ointment
	Pressure bandage	Apply new dressing
	Seek medical attention	

CARING FOR BURNS

- Cool the burned area.
- Cover the burned area.
- Minimize shock.
- Call EMS personnel for serious burns.

TM32

SIGNALS OF MUSCULOSKELETAL INJURIES

Common Signals

Pain

Swelling

Deformity

Discoloration

Limited use of body part

Signals of Serious Injury

Inability to use or move body part

Bone protruding from wound

Grating bones

Snapping or popping sound

Cause of injury

GENERAL CARE FOR MUSCULOSKELETAL INJURIES

- Rest
- Ice
- Elevation
- Immobilization

TM34

SERIOUS HEAD AND SPINE INJURIES

Signals

Altered consciousness

Severe pain/pressure

Loss of sensation/movement in extremities

Blood/fluids in the ears/nose

Serious bleeding

Seizures

Impaired breathing/vision

Nausea/vomiting

Persistent headache

Loss of balance

Care

Minimize movement.

Maintain an open airway.

Monitor consciousness and breathing.

Control bleeding.

Maintain normal body temperature.

Monitor vital signs.

Minimize shock.

SERIOUS CHEST INJURY

Signals

Difficulty breathing

Severe pain

Discoloration

Deformity

Coughing up blood

Object penetrating chest

"Sucking" sound when breathing

Care

Position the person to aid breathing.

If the ribs are broken, bind arm to injured side.

Cover sucking chest wound.

Call EMS.

TM36

SERIOUS ABDOMINAL INJURY

Signals

Nausea/vomiting

Thirst

Rigid abdomen

Weakness

Organs protruding from abdomen

Care

General Care:

Position victim on back.

Bend knees slightly.

Seek medical attention.

Minimize shock.

Open wound care:

Do not put pressure on protruding organs or try to put them back inside.

Cover loosely with moist, clean dressing.

Cover dressing with plastic wrap.

SERIOUS PELVIC INJURY

Signals

Nausea/vomiting

Thirst

Rigid abdomen

Weakness

Organs protruding from abdomen

Loss of sensation/movement in the legs

Pain

Care

Minimize movement.

Control bleeding.

Call EMS.

TM38

SERIOUS EXTREMITY INJURY

Signals

Pain

Tenderness

Swelling

Discoloration

Deformity

Loss of sensation/movement

Cool to the touch

Severe external bleeding

Care

Immobilize the injured area (splint).

Apply ice.

Call EMS.

SCENARIO 1

At work, you are summoned to assist another employee who has been injured in an 8-foot fall from a ladder. As you arrive, you see the person lying on the ground. She is crying and moaning in pain. A bystander says that she landed on her back. The victim has not moved from this position. She says that she has tingling and numbness in her legs and feet and pain in her back. She also has a 2-inch laceration on the side of her head. You want to help. How do you proceed?

SCENARIO 2

You and a friend are driving home, and see a collision between a bicyclist and skateboarder. Both are thrown to the pavement. Both are conscious and in pain. The skateboarder was struck on the outside of his leg by the bike. The leg is bent, and his knee has an obvious deformity. The bicyclist was thrown over the handlebars, landing on her outstretched arms. She is bleeding from abrasions on both forearms and her wrist has an obvious deformity. You have a first aid kit in your car. You want to help. How do you proceed?

SCENARIO 3

You are coaching a Little League baseball team. The pitcher is struck with a line drive to the ankle. The pitcher falls to the ground. He is crying and in pain, unable to move the limb. Slight swelling and discoloration are already present. You are about three minutes away from the nearest hospital. The player's parents are not at the game. You want to help. How do you proceed?

SCENARIO 4

On a cool fall day, you and a group of friends are hiking through a state park. The terrain you have chosen is rough, with a few steep inclines. After you have been hiking about an hour, suddenly one of the hikers loses his footing and tumbles approximately 30 feet down a steep slope. He strikes several rocks along the way. You and another hiker are able to make your way down to the victim quickly and safely. The victim appears to have been temporarily unconscious. While he is now conscious, he is dazed and unsure of his surroundings. There is a large bruise on his forehead. He says that he cannot move one of his arms. His elbow is bruised, swollen, and bleeding. He also has a stick approximately four inches long and one inch wide impaled in his hand. You have first aid supplies in your backpack. You want to help. How do you proceed?

COMMON SUDDEN ILLNESSES

- Fainting
- Diabetic emergencies
- Seizures
- Stroke
- Poisoning
- Heart attack

FAINTING

Signals

Altered consciousness

Shock-like signals

Ill feeling/appearance

Care

Position person on a flat surface.

Elevate legs.

Check ABCs.

Loosen clothing.

Call EMS.

DIABETIC EMERGENCY

Signals

Altered consciousness

Rapid breathing

Rapid pulse

Ill feeling/appearance

Care

Monitor ABCs.

Do a secondary survey. (Determine if victim is a diabetic.)

Conscious victim:

Give victim substance with sugar.

Unconscious victim:

Do not give anything by mouth.

Maintain normal body temperature.

Call EMS.

LYNNE RUSH

Answer Key: ARC First Aid—Responding to Emergencies Exam B

Question	a	b	c	d
1.		b	c	d
2.	a	b	●	d
3.	a	b	c	●
4.		b	c	d
5.	a	●	c	d
6.		b	c	d
7.	a	b	c	●
8.	a	b	●	d
9.		b	c	d
10.	a	b	c	●
11.	a	b	●	d
12.		b	c	d
13.	a	b	●	d
14.	a	b	c	●
15.	a	●	c	d
16.	a	b	c	●
17.	a	b	●	d
18.		b	c	d
19.	a	●	c	d
20.		b	c	d
21.	a	●	c	d
22.		b	c	d
23.	a	b	●	d
24.	a	b	c	●
25.		b	c	d
26.	a	b	c	●
27.	a	●	c	d
28.	a	b	●	d
29.	a	●	c	d
30.	a	b	●	d
31.	a	b	c	●
32.		b	c	d
33.	a	b	c	●
34.	a	●	c	d
35.	a	b	c	●
36.	a	b	c	●
37.	a	●	c	d
38.	a	b	c	●
39.	●	b	c	d
40.	a	b	●	d
41.	●	b	c	d
42.	a	b	c	●
43.	a	b	●	d
44.	a	b	c	●
45.	●	b	c	d
46.	a	b	●	d
47.	a	●	c	d
48.	●	b	c	d
49.	a	b	●	d
50.	a	b	c	●
51.	a	b	●	d
52.	a	b	c	●
53.	●	b	c	d
54.	a	b	c	●
55.	a	b	●	d
56.	a	b	c	●
57.	a	b	●	d
58.	a	b	c	●
59.	●	b	c	d
60.	a	b	c	●
61.	●	b	c	d
62.	a	b	c	●
63.	●	b	c	d
64.	a	b	c	●
65.	●	b	c	d
66.	a	b	c	●
67.	a	b	●	d
68.	a	b	c	●
69.	●	b	c	d
70.	a	b	c	●

LYNNE RUSH

Answer Key: ARC First Aid—Responding to Emergencies — Exam A

No.	a	b	c	d
1.	a	●	c	d
2.		b	c	d
3.	a	b	c	●
4.	a	b	●	d
5.	a	b	c	●
6.	a	●	c	d
7.	a	b	c	●
8.	a	b	●	d
9.		b	c	d
10.	a	b	●	d
11.	a	b	c	●
12.	a	●	c	d
13.	a	b	c	●
14.	a	b	●	d
15.	a	●	c	d
16.	a	b	●	d
17.		b	c	d
18.	a	●	c	d
19.	a	b	c	●
20.		b	c	d
21.	a	b	c	●
22.		b	c	d
23.	a	●	c	d
24.	a	b	c	●
25.	a	b	●	d
26.	a	b	c	●
27.	a	●	c	d
28.		b	c	d
29.	a	b	c	●
30.	a	●	c	d
31.	a	b	c	●
32.		b	c	d
33.	a	b	●	d
34.	a	●	c	d
35.	a	b	●	d
36.	a	b	●	d
37.	a	b	c	●
38.	a	●	c	d
39.	a	b	c	●
40.	a	b	●	d
41.	a	●	c	d
42.	●	b	c	d
43.	a	●	c	d
44.	a	b	c	●
45.	a	●	c	d
46.	●	b	c	d
47.	a	b	c	●
48.	a	b	●	d
49.	a	b	c	●
50.	a	b	●	d
51.	a	b	c	●
52.	a	●	c	d
53.	a	b	c	●
54.	●	b	c	d
55.	a	●	c	d
56.	●	b	c	d
57.	a	●	c	d
58.	a	b	●	d
59.	a	b	c	●
60.	a	b	●	d
61.	a	b	c	●
62.	a	b	●	d
63.	a	b	c	●
64.	●	b	c	d
65.	a	b	c	●
66.	a	●	c	d
67.	a	b	●	d
68.	a	●	c	d
69.	●	b	c	d
70.	a	b	●	d

SEIZURES

Signals

Altered consciousness

Blackouts

Uncontrollable muscle contractions

Ill feeling/appearance

Care

Protect from injury.

Monitor ABCs.

If fluid is present in mouth, position victim so fluid drains.

Do a secondary survey after a seizure.

Reassure the person.

Call EMS personnel if needed.

SEIZURES — WHEN TO CALL EMS

- Lasts more than a few minutes
- Repeated seizures
- Injury
- Uncertainty about cause
- Pregnant victim
- Diabetic victim
- Infant or child victim
- Occurs in water
- Victim remains unconscious

STROKE

Signals

Altered consciousness

Ill feeling/appearance

Sudden weakness/ numbness

Difficulty speaking

Blurred/dimmed vision

Unequal pupils

Sudden, severe headache

Care

Monitor ABCs.

Clear airway as needed.

Call EMS.

TM48

SIGNALS OF POISONING

The scene —

Odors

Flames/smoke

Open/empty/spilled containers

Overturned/damaged plants

The victim —

Nausea/vomiting

Chest/abdominal pain

Breathing difficulty

Altered consciousness

Seizures

Burns on/around mouth

CARING FOR MEDICAL EMERGENCIES

General Care

Maintain an open airway.

Monitor breathing, pulse, and consciousness.

Call EMS.

Position the victim comfortably.

Maintain normal body temperature.

Minimize shock.

Specific Care

Diabetic emergency—give sugar to conscious victim

Seizure—protect from injury

Poisoning—follow instructions from PCC/EMS

TM50

. 'ACTORS LEADING TO DRUG MISUSE/ ABUSE

- Lack of parental supervision
- Breakdown of family structure
- Wish to escape
- Availability of substances
- Peer pressure
- Low self-esteem
- Media glamorization

SCENARIO

A 25-year-old woman has several drinks at a party. She later says that she feels dizzy and nauseated. She goes into another room. Soon after, someone enters shouting that she has collapsed to the floor and is unconscious. Among the objects scattered on the floor from her open purse are several containers of pills. One is marked "Valium." You want to help. How would you proceed?

FACTORS AFFECTING BODY TEMPERATURE

- Air temperature
- Humidity
- Wind
- Clothing
- Activity
- Fluid intake
- Body adaptability

FACTORS AFFECTING RISK OF HEAT-RELATED AND COLD-RELATED ILLNESS

- Age
- Strenuous activity
- Predisposing health problems

SIGNALS OF HEAT–RELATED EMERGENCIES

Heat Cramps	Heat Exhaustion	Heat Stroke
Heavy Sweating	Shocklike —	Sweating stops
Rapid onset	Dizziness/weakness	Rapid rise in body temperature
Pain	Cool/moist skin	Altered consciousness
Muscle spasms	Nausea	Convulsions
		Body systems fail

CARING FOR HEAT-RELATED EMERGENCIES

Cool the victim —

- Remove from hot environment.
- Give cool water if conscious.
- Loosen/remove clothing.
- Apply wet towels/cold packs.
- Fan.

Call EMS

COLD-RELATED EMERGENCIES

	Signals	Care
Frostbite	Cold skin Discoloration	Handle gently. Warm in 100°–105° F water. Bandage loosely.
Hypothermia	Shivering Numbness Apathy Altered consciousness	Remove wet clothing. Gradually rewarm — Use dry blankets/clothing. Move to warm location. Give warm liquid. Call EMS.

SCENARIO

Twenty-year-old Todd Wilson is working for his uncle, remodeling, during the summer. He is putting fiberglass insulation in an attic. He is wearing long pants, a long-sleeved shirt, goggles, a face mask, and a hat to protect himself from contact with the fiberglass.

Outdoor temperatures have been running about 90° F, and this day is exceptionally humid as well. Todd had hoped to have finished this job the evening before, but was unable to get to it until noon. He expects that it will take about 4½ hours.

Because Todd is in a hurry, he is working quickly to complete the job. He thinks he may be able to save some time if he does not take any breaks. About two hours later, drenched with sweat, Todd starts to feel dizzy, weak, and nauseated. He barely has the energy to get down from the attic. How could Todd have prevented the heat-related emergency?

SCENARIO 1

For several hours, your 60-year-old uncle has been complaining of indigestion while at your home for a seafood cookout. He now states that he has severe stomach pain and is nauseated. He attributes this pain and nausea to the food he ate. You notice that his skin is rather pale, he is breathing rapidly, and he looks ill. You want to help. How do you proceed?

SCENARIO 2

An elderly neighbor is walking in front of your home. You notice him lose his balance and collapse to the ground. He is not fully conscious. His eyes are open and the left side of his face appears to be drooping. The victim is making mumbling sounds, but you cannot tell what he is saying. Suddenly, he begins to vomit. You want to help. How do you proceed?

SCENARIO 3

It is late afternoon, and your team is finishing its third match of the volleyball tournament on the beach. It has been a really hot day, with temperatures in the 90s. Suddenly, a teammate collapses. She does not appear to be fully conscious but is breathing rapidly. You notice her skin is very warm, sunburned, and moist. Her pulse is very fast. She is unable to get up from the ground. You want to help. How do you proceed?

SCENARIO 4

A dangerous ritual is about to begin —21 drinks for the 21st birthday. A group of close friends has gathered for a special party for the "birthday boy." Everyone knows it is a dangerous game, but because each of these friends went through it, they believe it is a rite of passage into adulthood. The activities begin, and the guest of honor is soon "chugging" beers and downing shots of liquor at a rapid pace. Two hours after the drinking began, you arrive at the party. The guest of honor is vomiting violently in the bathroom. He slumps to the floor and begins violent convulsions, followed by unconsciousness. He seems to stop breathing and then takes a deep breath. You are summoned to help. How do you proceed?

BASIC GUIDELINES FOR MOVING A VICTIM

- Move only if able.
- Bend at knees.
- Lift with legs, not with back.
- Take short steps.
- Move forward.
- Look where you are going.
- Protect victim.

CONSIDERATIONS FOR MOVING A VICTIM

- Danger at the scene
- Victim's size
- Rescuer's ability
- Assistance available
- Victim's condition

WATER SAFETY

- Respect the water.
- Supervise children.
- Wear flotation devices.
- Swim with a buddy.
- Swim in a supervised area.
- Avoid impairing substances.

SCENARIO 1

You are driving home with a friend at rush hour and witness an automobile collision involving one vehicle that has a struck a guard rail head-on. The car is still running. The driver did not have on a safety belt and struck the steering column. He is seated behind the steering wheel, conscious and complaining of chest and abdominal pain. The other passenger also was not wearing a safety belt. She is lying motionless, facedown on the floor of the vehicle. You see blood around her body. She is unconscious and not breathing. You are unsure if she has a pulse. How do you proceed?

SCENARIO 2

There is a chemical explosion at an industrial plant. A worker nearby has been injured. She has severe burns on her face, neck, chest, and arms. She has walked into another room away from the explosion and collapsed to the floor. She is conscious with no other apparent injuries. There is danger of another explosion. You and a co-worker are close by and available to come to her aid. How do you proceed?

FOUR BASIC FOOD GROUPS

- Carbohydrates
- Dairy products
- Proteins
- Fruits and vegetables

CARDIOVASCULAR FITNESS

Helps you —

- Cope with stress.
- Control weight.
- Fight off infections.
- Improve self-esteem.
- Sleep better.

TM68

GUIDELINES FOR ALCOHOL CONSUMPTION

- Limit drinking to one drink or less per hour.
- Have nonalcoholic beverages available.
- Do not drink if depressed or angry.
- Do not drink before a party.
- Have food available.
- Avoid drinking games.
- Have designated drivers.

SCENARIO 1

As you are being escorted to your table in a restaurant, a man hastens by you, coughing repeatedly. A few minutes later, the maitre d' rushes in, asking for assistance. You overhear him and decide to help. As you are led outside, you see a man lying facedown on the sidewalk, not moving. Others have gathered around, but no one is doing anything. You recognize the man as the one who rushed past you in the restaurant. How do you proceed?

SCENARIO 2

Your younger sister is taking riding lessons at a nearby ranch. You go with her one day to watch her practice. Today she is riding a different horse from the one she normally rides. Suddenly, she is thrown from the horse. She falls flat on her back, striking her head on the ground. She lies motionless on the ground. The horse trots nearby. Her riding instructor is present to help. How do you proceed?

SCENARIO 3

You and your brother have just finished some yard work. Your brother goes inside to clean up. While still outside, you hear the sound of a chain saw nearby. You remember a neighbor saying that he was going to remove a large, dead tree in his yard. You decide to go over and see what is going on. Before you get far, you hear the sound of cracking wood, then you suddenly hear the saw stop, followed immediately by screams. You rush to your neighbor's yard. You see your neighbor sitting on the ground. Blood is pouring from a deep, large laceration just above his knee. Your neighbor is already "white as a ghost," is still screaming, and appears panic stricken. He is not making any effort to control the bleeding. You are alone with him. How do you proceed?

SCENARIO 4

In the middle of a pick-up basketball game at a local playground, two players go up for a rebound. As they collide, they both lose their balance and fall to the ground. As one player lands, she twists her ankle violently. The other player falls on her outstretched arm and appears to have injured her wrist and forearm. Both victims are conscious and moaning. How do you proceed?

Index First Aid—Responding to Emergencies

Notes

Notes

Notes

Notes